Practical
BIOCHEMISTRY
with Clinical Correlation

for MBBS Students

Covers all Practicals Prescribed by Medical Council of India (MCI) under Competency Based Undergraduate Curriculum for the Indian Medical Graduate

Practical BIOCHEMISTRY with Clinical Correlation

for MBBS Students

Covers all Practicals Prescribed by Medical Council of India (MCI) under Competency Based Undergraduate Curriculum for the Indian Medical Graduate

Poonam Agrawal MD (Biochemistry)

Professor and Head
Department of Biochemistry
Dr Baba Saheb Ambedkar Medical College and Hospital
New Delhi

CBS Publishers & Distributors Pvt Ltd

New Delhi • Bengaluru • Chennai • Kochi • Kolkata • Mumbai
Hyderabad • Jharkhand • Nagpur • Patna • Pune • Uttarakhand

Disclaimer

Science and technology are constantly changing fields. New research and experience broaden the scope of information and knowledge. The author has tried her best in giving information available to her while preparing the material for this book. Although all efforts have been made to ensure optimum accuracy of the material, yet it is quite possible some errors might have been left uncorrected. The publisher, the printer and the author will not be held responsible for any inadvertent errors or inaccuracies.

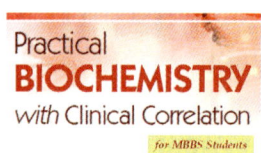

ISBN: 978-93-88178-89-1

Copyright © Author and Publisher

First Edition: 2021

All rights reserved. No part of this book may be reproduced or transmitted in any form or by any means, electronic or mechanical, including photocopying, recording, or any information storage and retrieval system without permission, in writing, from the author and the publisher.

Published by Satish Kumar Jain and Produced by Varun Jain for

CBS Publishers & Distributors Pvt Ltd
4819/XI Prahlad Street, 24 Ansari Road, Daryaganj, New Delhi 110 002, India.
Ph: 011-23289259, 23266861, 23266867   Fax: 011-23243014   Website: www.cbspd.com
e-mail: delhi@cbspd.com; cbspubs@airtelmail.in.
Corporate Office: 204 FIE, Industrial Area, Patparganj, Delhi 110 092
Ph: 011-4934 4934   Fax: 011-4934 4935   e-mail: publishing@cbspd.com; publicity@cbspd.com

Branches

- **Bengaluru:** Seema House 2975, 17th Cross, K.R. Road, Banasankari 2nd Stage, Bengaluru 560 070, Karnataka
  Ph: +91-80-26771678/79   Fax: +91-80-26771680   e-mail: bangalore@cbspd.com
- **Chennai:** 7, Subbaraya Street, Shenoy Nagar, Chennai 600 030, Tamil Nadu
  Ph: +91-44-26680620, 26681266   Fax: +91-44-42032115   e-mail: chennai@cbspd.com
- **Kochi:** 42/1325, 1326, Power House Road, Opp KSEB, Power House, Ernakulam 682 018, Kochi, Kerala, India
  Ph: +91-484-4059061-67   Fax: +91-484-4059065   e-mail: kochi@cbspd.com
- **Kolkata:** 6/B, Ground Floor, Rameswar Shaw Road, Kolkata 700 014, West Bengal
  Ph: +91-33-22891126, 22891127, 22891128   e-mail: kolkata@cbspd.com
- **Mumbai:** 83-C, Dr E Moses Road, Worli, Mumbai 400018, Maharashtra
  Ph: +91-22-24902340/41   Fax: +91-22-24902342   e-mail: mumbai@cbspd.com

Representatives

• Hyderabad	0-9885175004	• Jharkhand	0-9811541605	• Nagpur	0-9421945513
• Patna	0-9334159340	• Pune	0-9623451994	• Uttarakhand	0-9716462459

Printed at Goyal Offset Works (P) Limited, India

to
My Husband
Dr Mohit Agarwal

Preface

This book is based on Competency Based Medical Education [CBME] curriculum implemented by MCI. The focus of current CBME curriculum is on developing the competencies in medical students along with clinical correlation of subject biochemistry. According to current guidelines, the practical in biochemistry in medical college should be relevant in clinical diagnosis and management of the patient.

Old and obsolete practicals like gastric juice analysis, titrations, etc. have no role in current MBBS curriculum rather emphasis is on automated techniques, point of care testing and techniques and tools required in disease diagnosis. Accordingly these outdated techniques have been replaced by new state to art techniques and their application in clinical setting in relevant chapters.

I sincerely hope that this attempt to present the practicals in biochemistry for medical undergraduates in **conceptual, clinical and correlated fashion** will be appreciated by medical students and faculties.

Feedback and suggestions are welcome

Poonam Agrawal
drpoonam24agrawal@yahoo.com

Acknowledgements

First of all, I would like to thank almighty for giving me the dream and then the courage to work hard to fulfil it.

I thankfully acknowledge the love and belief of my dear students which has motivated me to write this to make their understanding of practical in subject easier.

I acknowledge the contribution of many of my colleagues and friends who have always encouraged me to do good work. This piece of work is also because of their encouragement and faith in me. I would like to mention some of them here

Dr Santosh Kumar, Professor and Head, Department of Biochemistry, Nalanda Medical College, Nalanda.

Dr Niket Verma, Assistant Professor, Department of Medicine, Army College of Medical Sciences, New Delhi.

A big thanks to the fabulous team at CBS Publishers & Distributors, especially to Mr YN Arjuna Senior Vice-President—Publishing, Editorial and Publicity, **Mrs Ritu Chawla** General Manager—Production, **Mr Vikrant Sharma** for the dedicated formatting, Mr Rohan Prasad (graphic artist), Mr Neeraj Prasad for cover design and to Mr Surendra Jha for the meticulous reading.

Words can't express the gratitude I feel toward my husband Dr Mohit Agarwal and my baby Misti for their unconditional support and tons of adjustments throughout this period when I was engrossed in writing this manuscript.

Poonam Agrawal

Contents

Preface vii

Section I: Laboratory Intruments and Biosafety

1. Commonly Used Laboratory Apparatus and Equipment — 3
2. Safe Laboratory Practice and Waste Disposal — 22

Section II: Qualitative Assessments

3. Analysis of Normal Urine for Its Constituents — 33
4. Analysis of Abnormal Constituents in the Urine and Their Clinical Correlation — 43

Section III: Quantitative Analysis

5. Colorimeter and Spectrophotometer: Principle and Their Functioning — 59
6. Estimation of Glucose in Serum and Other Biological Fluids — 66
7. Kidney Function Test: An Overview — 79
8. Estimation of Urea in Serum and Other Biological Fluids — 87
9. Estimation of Creatinine in Serum and Other Biological Fluids — 95
10. Estimation of Uric Acid in Serum — 104
11. Liver Function Test: An Overview — 110
12. Estimation of Bilirubin — 116
13. Estimation of AST/SGOT — 122
14. Estimation of SGPT (ALT) — 128
15. Estimation of ALP — 134
16. Estimation of Total Protein in Serum and Other Biological Fluids — 139
17. Estimation of Albumin in Serum and Calculation of A:G Ratio — 145
18. Estimation of Total Cholesterol — 150
19. Estimation of Triacylglycerol and HDL — 158
20. Estimation of Calcium — 162
21. Estimation of Phosphorus — 168

Section IV: Organ Function Tests

22. Thyroid, Pancreatic and Gastric Function Tests — 175

Section V: Clinical Lab Patient's Report Interpretation (Chart Discussion/Spotter)

23. Enzyme as a Marker of Disease — 187
24. Interpretation of Laboratory Result: Carbohydrate Metabolism — 193
25. Interpretation of Laboratory Result: Oral Glucose Tolerance Test (OGTT) — 199
26. Interpretation of Laboratory Result: Amino Acid Metabolism — 207
27. Interpretation of Laboratory Result: Lipid Metabolism — 213
28. Interpretation of Laboratory Result: Protein Metabolism — 217
29. Interpretation of Laboratory Result: Purine Nucleotide Metabolism — 224
30. Interpretation of Laboratory Result: Arterial Blood Gas (ABG) Analysis — 228
31. Cerebrospinal Fluid (CSF) — 234

Section VI: Vitamin and Mineral Deficiencies and Their Clinical Manifestation (Chart Discussion/Spotter)

32. Water-Soluble Vitamins — 241
33. Fat-Soluble Vitamins — 249
34. Minerals and Clinical Manifestation of Their Plasma Level Derangements — 255

Section VII: Techniques

35. Electrophoresis — 267
36. Chromatography — 276

Section I

Laboratory Instruments and Biosafety

1. Commonly Used Laboratory Apparatus and Equipment
2. Safe Laboratory Practice and Waste Disposal

CHAPTER

1

Commonly Used Laboratory Apparatus and Equipment

Competencies

BI 11.1: Describe commonly used laboratory apparatus and equipment.
BI 11.19: Outline the basic principles involved in the functioning of instruments commonly used in a biochemistry laboratory and their applications.
BI 11.16: Observe use of commonly used equipment/techniques in biochemistry.

Various instruments and equipment used in undergraduate biochemistry lab and clinical biochemistry lab are:
- Balances
- Magnetic stirrer
- Centrifuge
- Hot air oven
- Incubator
- Water bath
- Desiccator
- pH meter
- Thermometer
- Various glasswares
- Semiautoanalyzer
- Fully autoanalyzer
- Electrophoresis (described in Chapter 36)
- Chromatography (described in Chapter 37)
- Colorimeter/photometer/spectrophotometer (described in Chapter 5)

There are many instruments which are being used in different biochemistry lab for teaching and diagnostic purposes. Their description is given in this chapter along with the principle of their functioning and the application.

Balances

It is important to prepare reagents and standard solution with accurate measurement of various chemicals. For this purpose, the instrument used is "Balance".

There are various types of balances used in biochemistry lab. They are:
a. Physical/mechanical balance
b. Electronic balance

Physical (Mechanical) Balance

- It is rather a crude equipment which is used for measuring chemicals which are needed for making qualitative reagents and where larger amount of chemical need to be measured.
- They are double-pan balances where on one side known weight is kept and on other side chemical to be measured is equated.
- The weight which can be measured in this instrument vary from **1 mg to 1000 g**.
- Physical balance may be **open** two-pan balance or it may be a balance in **closed** compartment (Fig. 1.1).

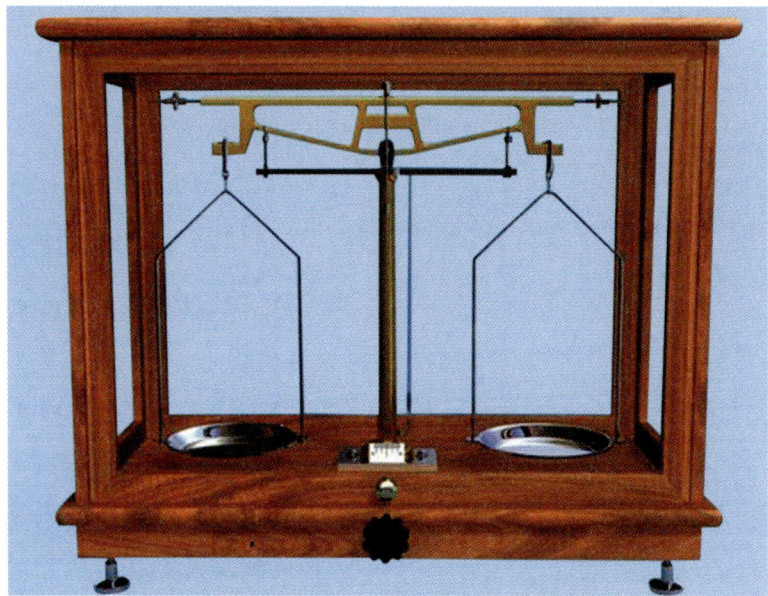

Fig. 1.1: Physical balance in closed compartment

Electronic Balances

They are more accurate and are being preferred because of accuracy and ease of operation. They are **single pan balances** which operate on **principle of electromagnetic force** which counterbalance the weighed sample mass. It measures rather smaller amount compared to physical balance. The weight which can be measured ranges from **1 mg to 100 g**.

Facility of **"taring"** in electronic balances makes the measurement easier as because of it the weight of container is adjusted by the machine itself (Fig. 1.2).

Magnetic Stirrer

This is used for thorough mixing of solutes in the solution to make a homogenous mixture. An iron capsule is placed in the vessel containing solution and then this vessel is placed on the pan of magnetic stirrer plate which is built to provide rotating magnetic field.

Movement of iron capsule in the solution on switching on the instrument mixes the solution completely as to provide the homogenous mixture (Fig. 1.3).

Commonly Used Laboratory Apparatus and Equipment

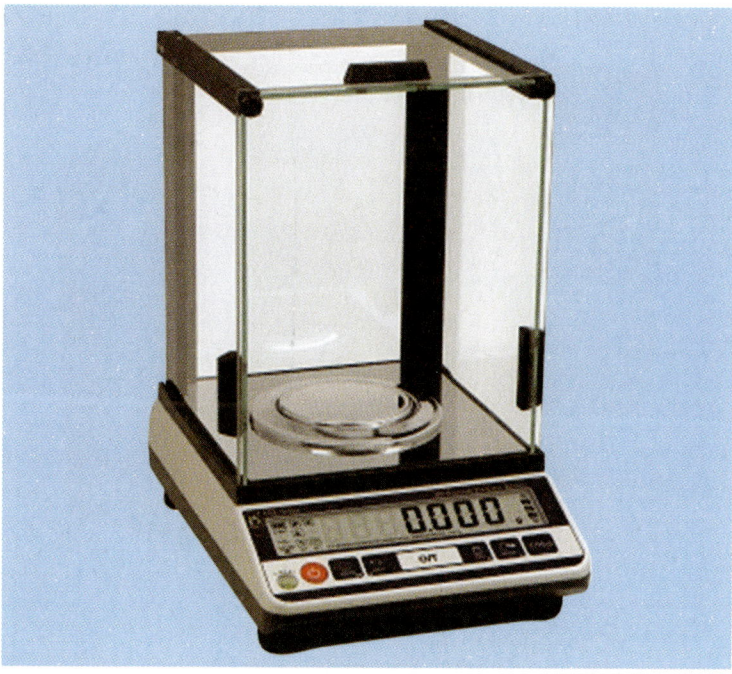

Fig. 1.2: Electronic balance

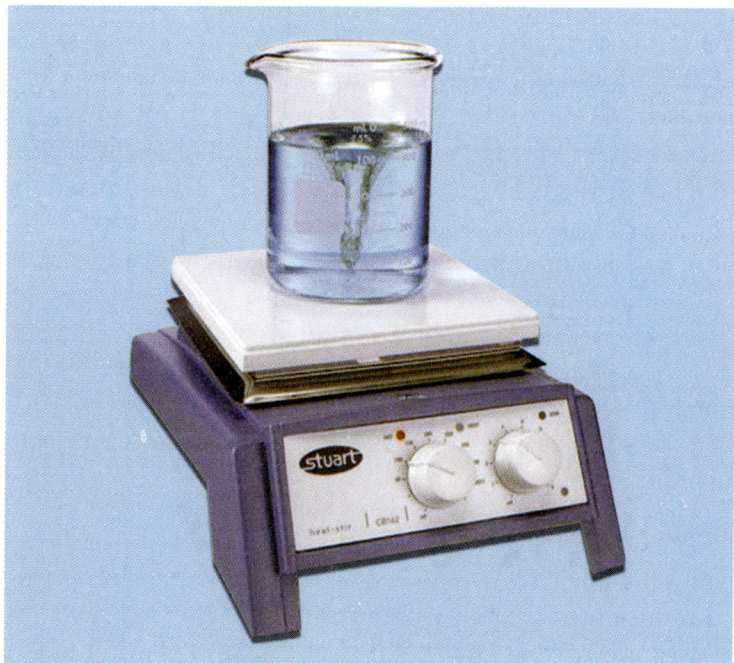

Fig. 1.3: Magnetic stirrer

Centrifuge

This instrument is commonly used in biochemistry lab to separate serum or plasma from whole blood and it also separates sediments in the urine (Fig. 1.4).

Centrifuge is based on the **principle of centrifugal force** which is used to separate solid matters from liquid suspension.

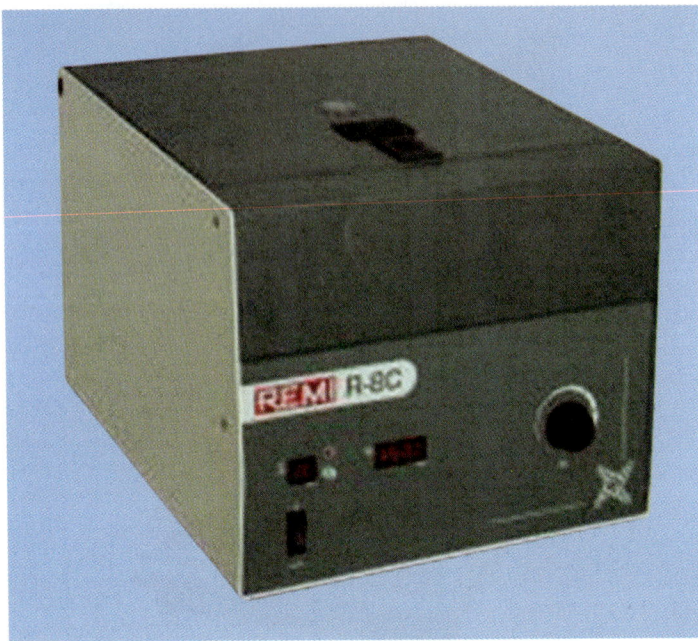

Fig. 1.4: Centrifuge

Centrifuge can be classified as:
a. Bench-top or floor model
b. With refrigeration and without refrigeration
c. Based on rotor design
d. Based on maximum speed which can be attained (normal or ultracentrifuge)

Rotor is the component of the centrifuge machine which is holding the tubes or vacutainers. Based on rotor design, we have two types of centrifuge:
- Horizontal rotor type (swing out head)
- Fixed angle rotor type (angle head)

Fixed angle rotor type of centrifuge can be operated at high speed compare to horizontal rotor type.

This is the reason that lesser air friction is generated in fixed angle type resulting in lesser heat production. In swing out rotor type of centrifuge, more air friction results in more heat production, hence it cannot be operated at very high speed.

Principle of Centrifuge Machine

Key factor in separating the particulate matter from liquid suspension is the **relative centrifugal force (RCF)** which is represented by following formula

$$RCF = R \times (RPM)^2 \times 118 \times 10^{-7}$$

R is the rotating radius of the rotor which means the radius of rotating path from the central axis.

RPM (revolution per minute): It is the number of revolutions of rotor in a minute. It can be programmed in the centrifuge.

Ultracentrifuge: The centrifuge which can be operated at **very high speed (1,00,000 RPM)** is known as ultracentrifuge.

Hot Air Oven

It is the equipment which produces dry heat in its internal chamber, the temperature may go up to 250°C. These were originally developed by Pasteur. It has double-walled insulation which conserves the heat (Fig. 1.5).

This is used for:
1. Drying of the glassware
2. Heating the chemicals wherever required
3. Dry sterilization of glassware (in microbiological experiments), metal equipment, swabs, etc.

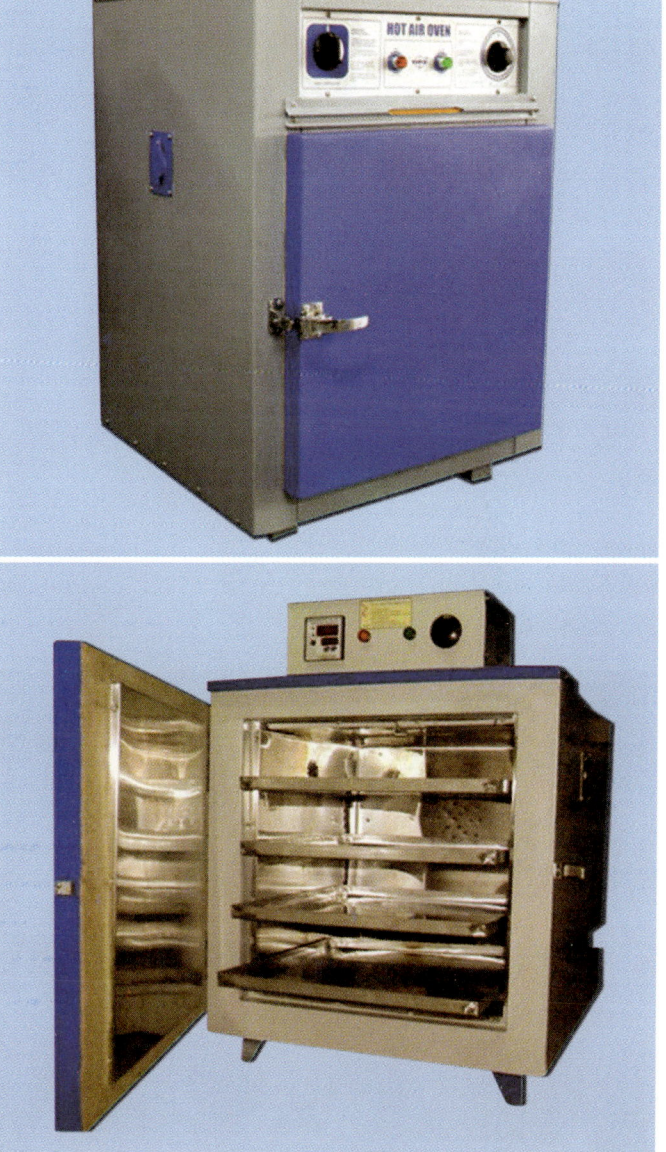

Fig. 1.5: Hot air oven

Incubator

It is an instrument which is capable of maintaining desired temperature, humidity, oxygen and CO_2 in the atmosphere inside (Fig. 1.6).

It is mainly used in microbiology for culture of organism under specified conditions. In biochemistry, incubator is important to incubate the reaction mixture at specific temperature for set duration which depends upon the method adopted for assessment.

Here the temperature may go up to 60–65°C, never beyond 100°C.

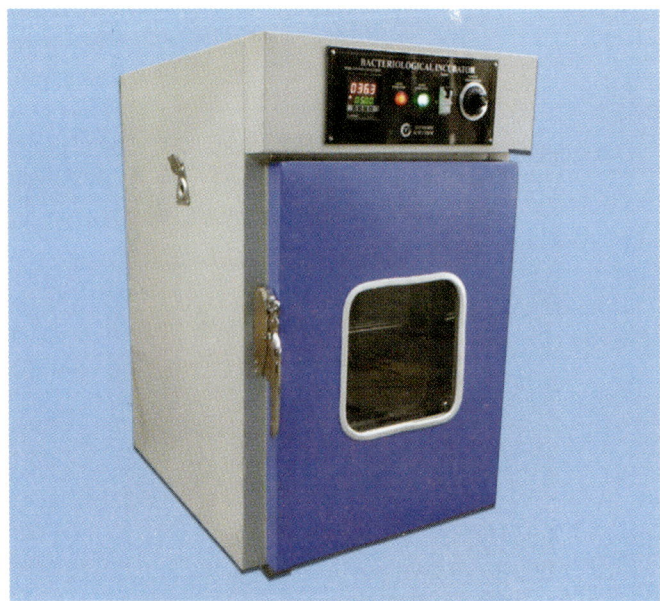

Fig. 1.6: Incubator

Water Bath

This equipment has water filled in it, the temperature of which can be controlled by adjustment (Fig. 1.7).

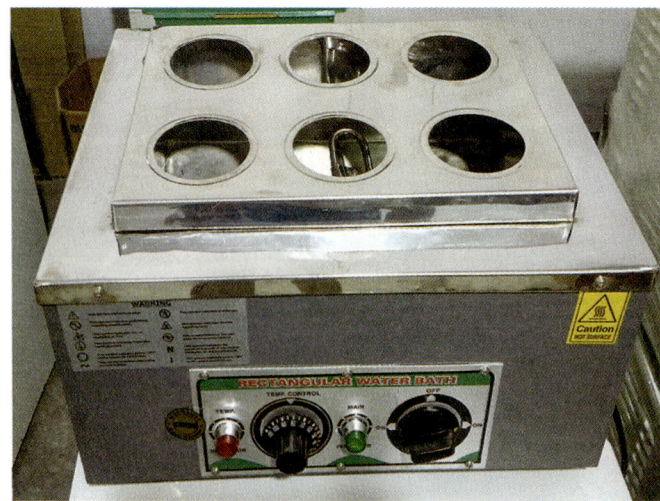

Fig. 1.7: Water bath

This is used for various experiments where a specified temperature is used for heating the reaction mixture. It is commonly used in medical undergraduate practicals where heating of solution is desired. In this equipment, sample can be heated at constant temperature over a prolonged period of time.

Desiccator and Desiccants

Desiccants are hygroscopic substances which absorb water from atmosphere and from various other hydrated substances. In other words, desiccants are **drying agents**. In biochemical lab, we need to remove moisture from many chemicals before using them for analytical purpose, for that purpose these chemicals are kept in contact with desiccants in a closed, airtight chamber which has a lid with a lubricated seal known as desiccator (Fig. 1.8).

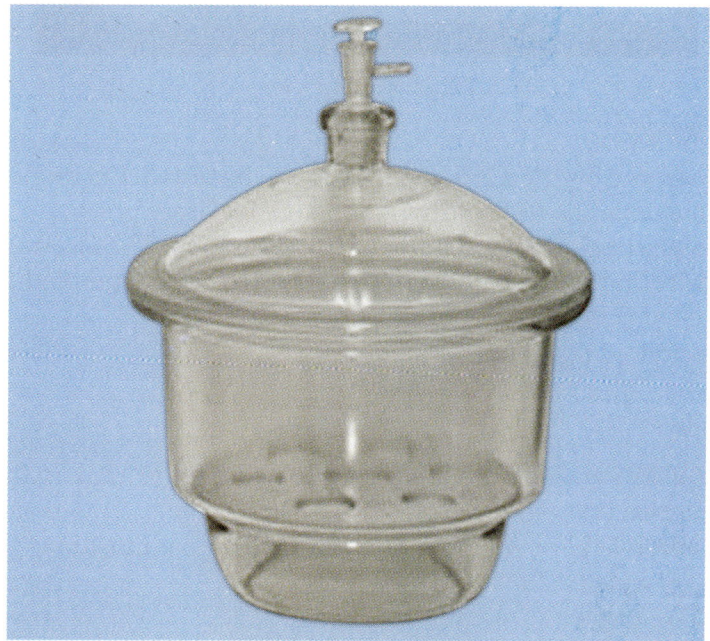

Fig. 1.8: Desiccator

pH Meter

What is pH?

pH of a solution is negative logarithm of the hydrogen ion concentration. It can be expressed as:

$$pH = 1/\log_{10}(H^+)$$

As stated in equation above, pH of a solution is inversely proportional to its hydrogen ion concentration. Normal pH of some important biological fluids in human is enumerated below:

- Plasma = 7.35 to 7.45 [Mean = 7.4]
- Urine = 6.5
- CSF = 7.32
- Gastric juice = 1.0 to 2.0

pH meter: pH meter is a reliable and convenient method of measuring the pH of a solution. The pH meter measures the difference in electric potential between a pH electrode and a reference electrode, and so the pH meter is sometimes referred to as a **"potentiometric pH meter"** (Fig. 1.9).

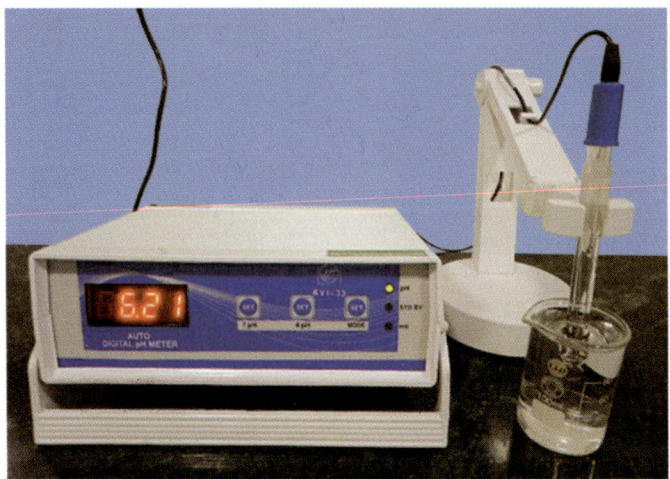

Fig. 1.9: pH meter

Principle of its Functioning

The electrodes, or probes, are inserted into the solution to be tested. On immersion in the solution to be tested, hydrogen ions in the test solution exchange for other positively charged ions on the glass bulb, creating an electrochemical potential across the bulb. The electronic amplifier detects the difference in electrical potential between the two electrodes generated in the measurement and converts the potential difference to pH units.

This instrument has following components in it:
- Glass electrode
- Calomel electrode

Glass electrode: It has a thin-walled bulb which is filled with 0.1 M HCl. In this HCl, a silver wire coated with AgCl is dipped (Fig. 1.10).

The hydrogen ion selective glass membrane has following composition:
- CaO: 6%
- N_2O: 22%
- SiO_2: 72%

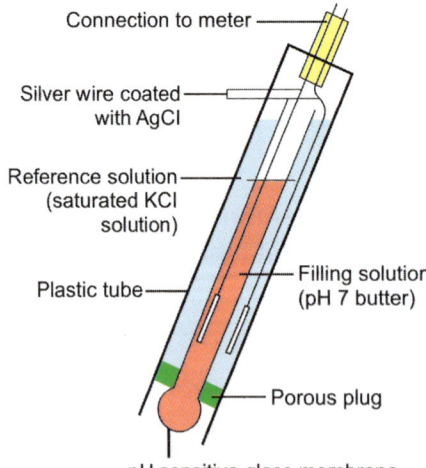

Fig. 1.10: pH meter (glass electrode)

Calomel electrode: It consists of glass tube which is filled with saturated solution of KCl and KCl porous material is plugged at the tip. In this solution, mercuric-mercurous electrode is dipped, the tip of which has porous plug of mercury calomel paste.

Combined electrode: In actual instrument, reference electrode and measuring electrodes are combined.

Thermometer

Many analytical reactions require an optimal temperature at which they occur. Enzymatic reactions specially need precise control of temperature. Many other reactions in biochemical system occur at wide range of temperature. In addition to this, many instruments like laboratory refrigerator, incubators, hot air oven, etc. need to have temperature display to monitor their accurate functioning.

Thermometer is the device which is used to monitor the temperature of the environment. It may be an integral part of the instrument or can be placed in the device for this purpose. Three major types of thermometers are:

1. Liquid in glass thermometer
2. Electronic thermometer (thermistor)
3. Digital thermometer

Liquid in glass thermometer has coloured liquid or mercury which is filled in glass or transparent plastic stem with bulb at one of its ends. Stem is graduated to record the temperature **(Fig. 1.11)**.

In era of automation, electronic thermometer (thermistor) is incorporated in many devices which give accurate and fast reading.

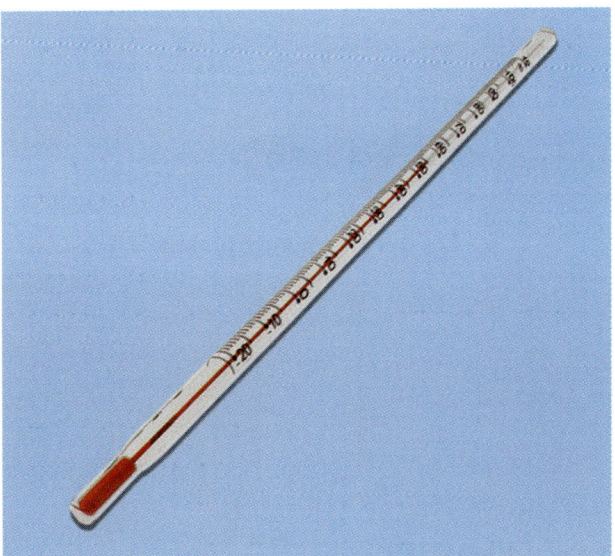

Fig. 1.11: Thermometer

Glasswares

A number of glasswares are used in biochemistry laboratories. The glassware which is used to transfer the liquid may be the one which is to contain (TC) or to deliver (TD) type based on how accurately the specified volume of liquid is transferred.

Various glasswares are described below:
- Flask
- Griffin beaker

- Graduated cylinder
- Pipettes
- Burets

Flask

Volumetric flask: This flask has round lower portion with flat bottom, along with a long narrow neck where calibrated line is marked. This kind of flask is used to prepare a specific volume of reagent (Fig. 1.12).

Erlenmeyer flask: This flask has wide bottom with narrow neck and is designed to hold different volumes of liquid. For this purpose, there is marking of various volumes on its wall (Fig. 1.13).

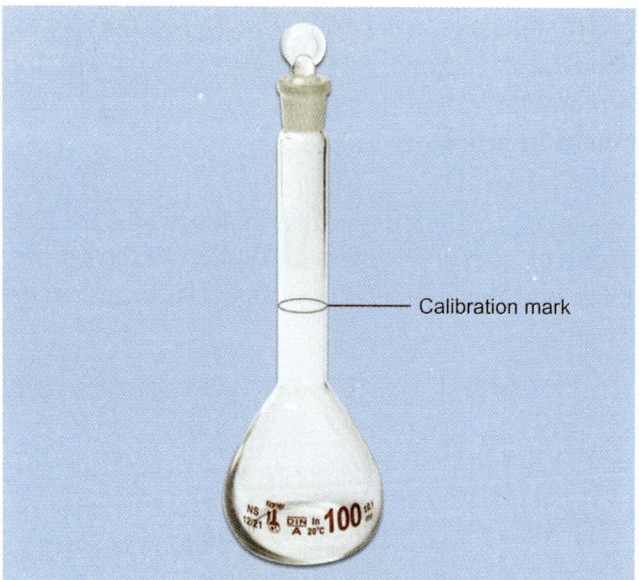

Fig. 1.12: Volumetric flask

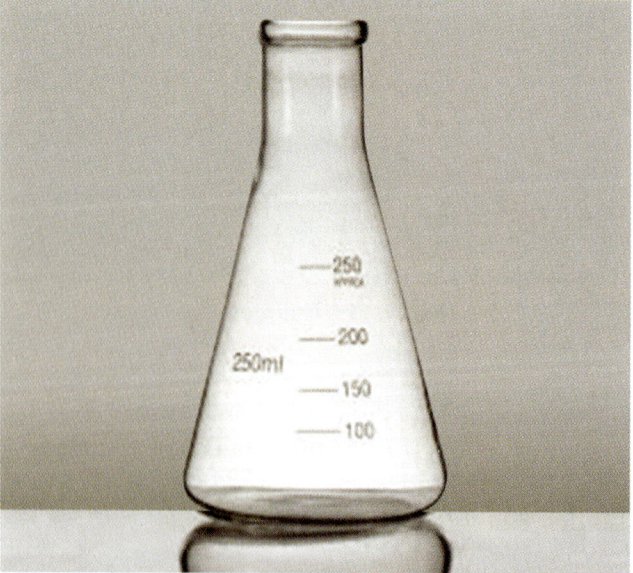

Fig. 1.13: Erlenmeyer flask

Griffin Beaker

It has flat bottom and straight wall with wide opening. It has marking on its side wall and can be used to store various volumes of solution (Fig. 1.14).

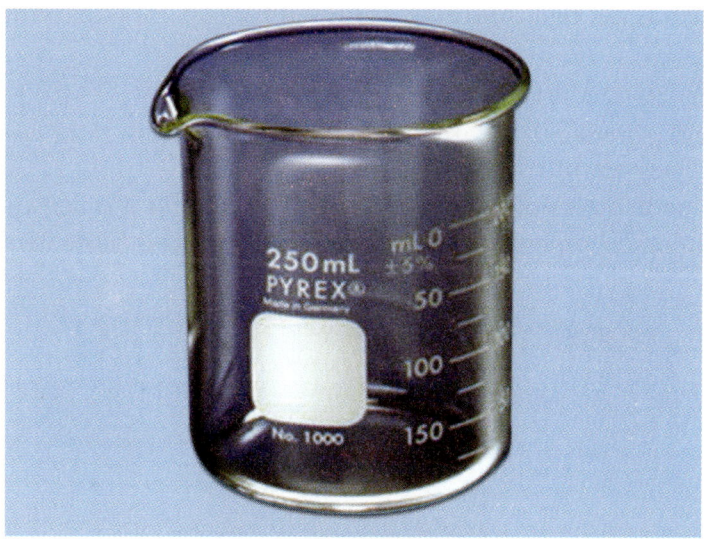

Fig. 1.14: Griffin beaker

Graduated Cylinder

These are cylinders having long stem and round or octagonal base. The side wall has markings of various volumes and this is used to measure volume of the reagent. It is available in various capacities from 10 to 2000 mL (Fig. 1.15).

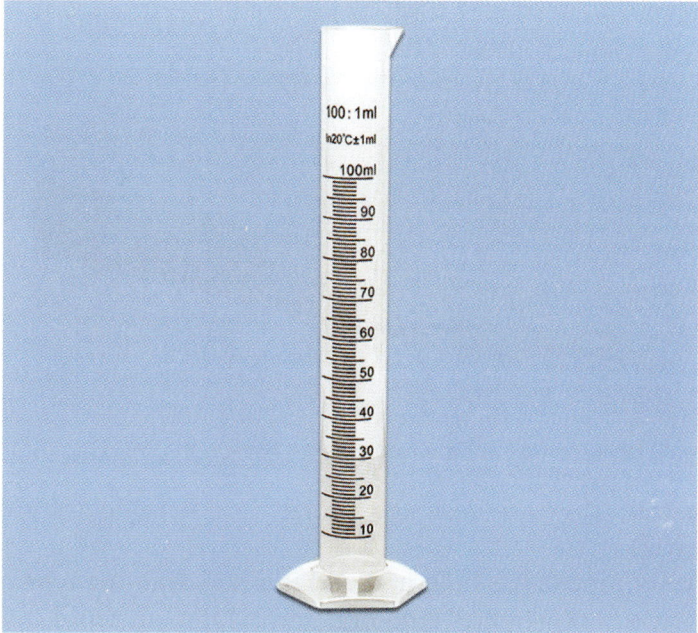

Fig. 1.15: Graduated cylinder

Pipette

Pipettes may be **TC (to contain) or TD (to deliver)** type depending upon whether it is delivering the exact specified volume or not as explained above.

Depending upon the draining characteristic, pipette may be **self-draining type or blowout type. Blowout pipette has got two continuous rings at the top.** Pipettes without this marking are self-draining type.

There are two major classes of pipettes: Measuring (graduated) and transfer types.

Measuring (graduated) pipettes: They are designed to dispense different volumes for which they have markings on it. They are of two types:
1. *Mohr type*: Mohr pipette does not have graduations till tip and it is self-draining type.
2. *Serological type*: Serological pipette has graduation till tip and is blowout type (Fig. 1.16).

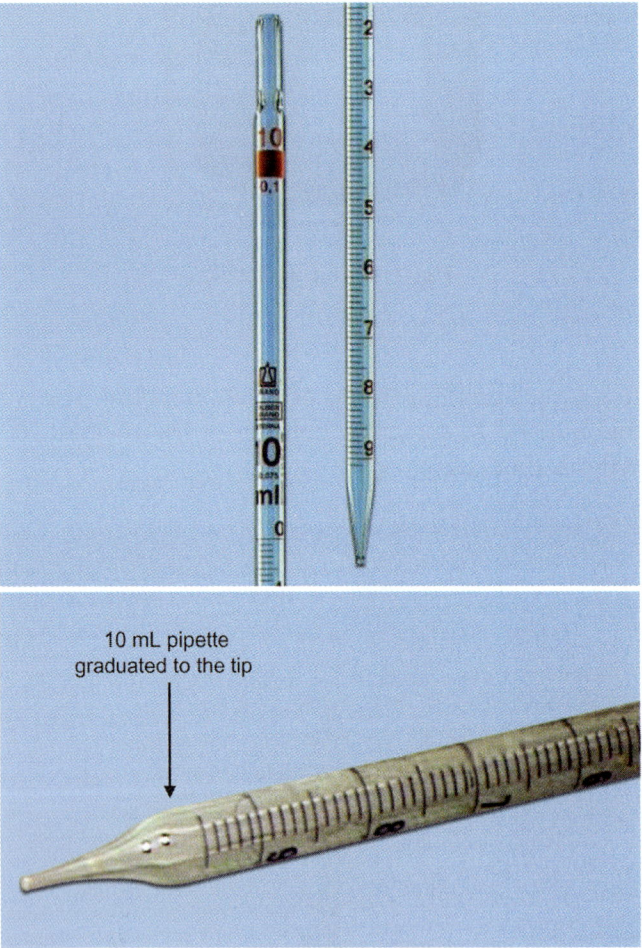

Fig. 1.16: Serological blowout pipette. Notice the marking till tip

Transfer type of pipettes: They are designed to deliver a specific volume alone. They are of following types (Fig. 1.17):
1. *Volumetric*: This type of pipette has bulb in it and it is self-draining type.
2. *Ostwald-Folin*: This type of pipette has bulb in it and is blowout type.
3. *Pasteur*: No calibration mark, not used for quantitative test (Fig. 1.18).

Commonly Used Laboratory Apparatus and Equipment

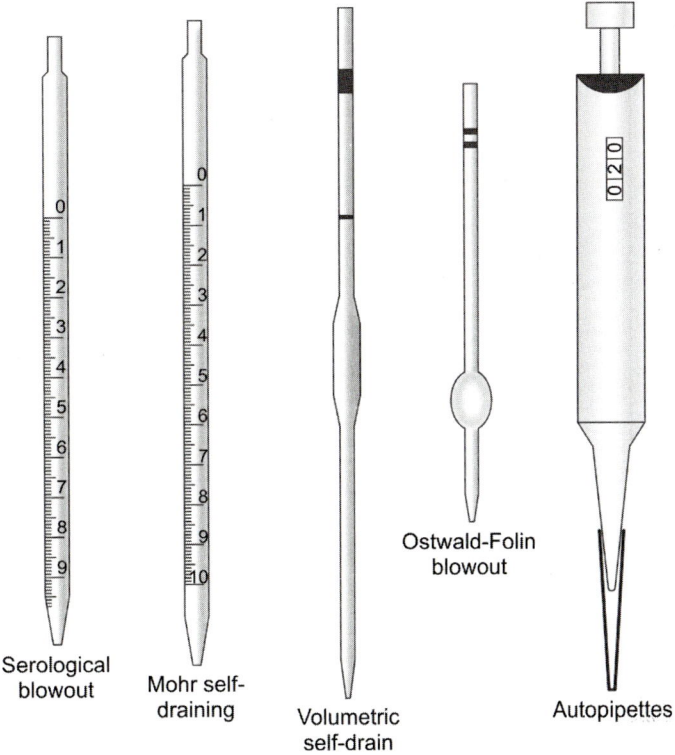

Fig. 1.17: Various types of pipettes

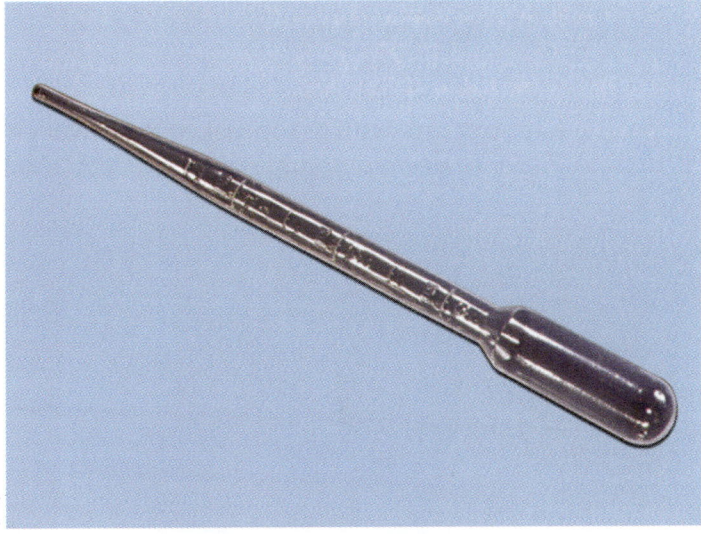

Fig. 1.18: Pasteur pipette

Nowadays **autopipettes** are used commonly to transfer volume less than 1 mL. They are easy to use and accuracy is high. They are of mainly two varieties: **Fixed volume and variable type.** Those which are designed to transfer volume of fluid less than 1 mL are called micropipettes and those which transfer larger volume of liquid are called **automatic macropipettes** (Fig. 1.19).

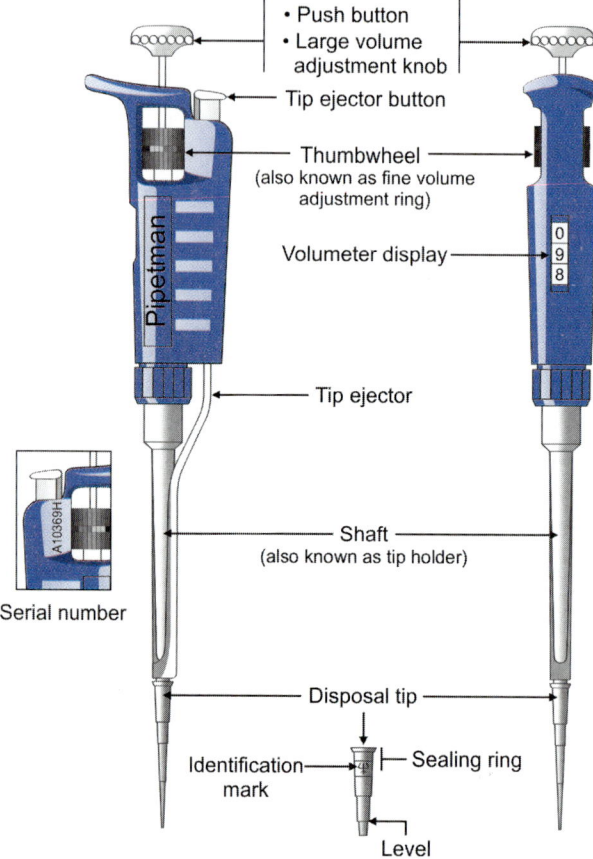

Fig. 1.19: Autopipette

Burets

It is long, graduated big pipette-like structure with a stopcock at the lower end. Its volume ranges from 25 to 100 mL. It is used to dispense desired volume of liquid drop by drop (Fig. 1.20).

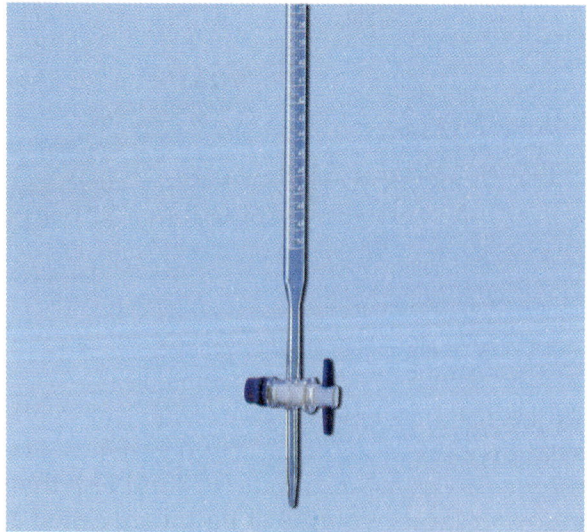

Fig. 1.20: Burets

Semiautoanalyzer

Principle and Functioning

Semiautomatic biochemistry analyzer is capable of performing routine biochemistry, hormonal assay, electrolytes, therapeutic drugs and drug-enzyme investigations. This instrument is based on principle of photometry described under colorimeter description in Chapter 5.

Semiautomated biochemistry analyzer is capable to perform tests on whole blood, serum, plasma, cerebrospinal fluid and urine as sample and it is suitable for small-sized laboratory (Fig. 1.21).

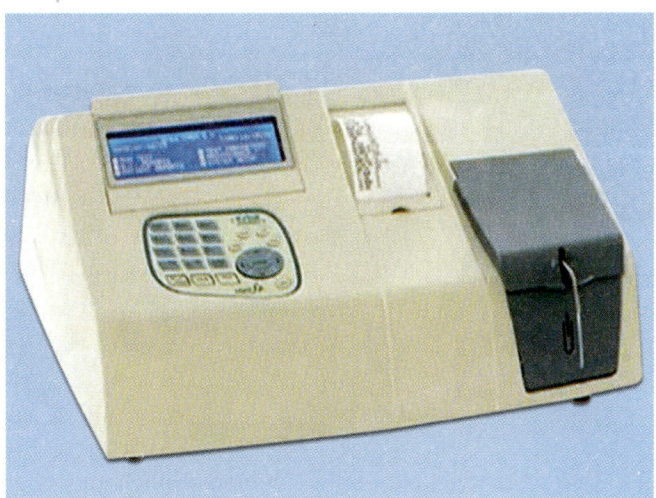

Fig. 1.21: Semiautoanalyzer

Fully Autoanalyzer

Principle and Functioning

The automatic biochemical analyzer has automated the sequence of operation processes which used to be conducted manually in past (Fig. 1.22).

It is based on colorimetric principle.

Important components of fully autoanalyzer are given in Fig. 1.23.

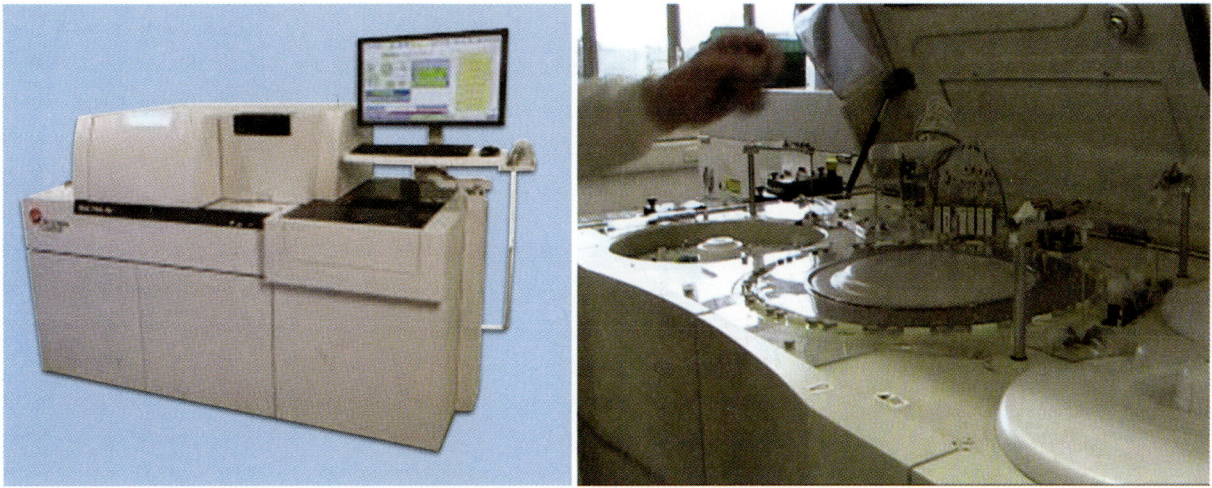

Fig. 1.22: Fully autoanalyzer

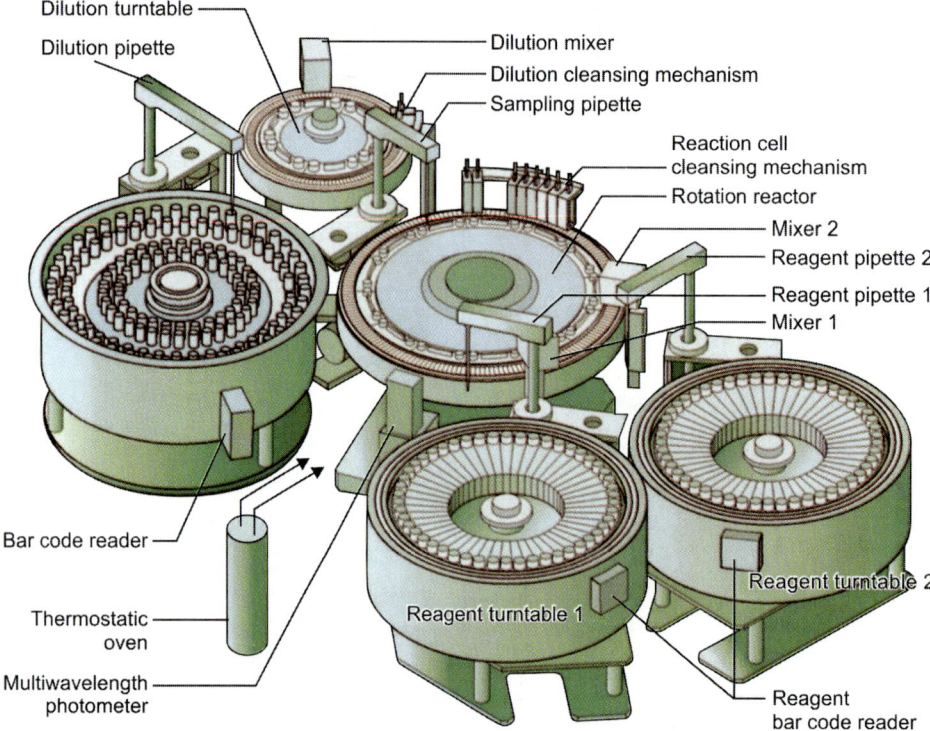

Fig. 1.23: Core components of fully automated biochemistry analyzer

Following are important parts in a fully autoanalyzer:
1. Reagent carousel
2. Sample compartment
3. Reaction cell
4. Sample probe (pipette)
5. Reagent probe (pipette)
6. Dilution pipette
7. Mixer

Commonly Used Laboratory Apparatus and Equipment

VIVA VOCE

Q1. How many types of balances are being used in biochemistry lab?
Ans. There are various types of balances used in biochemistry lab. They are:
a. Physical/mechanical balance
b. Electronic balance

Q2. What do you understand by term "Taring" in electronic balance?
Ans. Facility of "taring" in electronic balances makes the measurement easier as because of it the wait of container is adjusted by the machine itself.

Q3. What is magnetic stirrer and why it is used?
Ans. This is used for thorough mixing of solutes in the solution to make a homogenous mixture

Q4. How many variations of centrifuge you know?
Ans. Centrifuge can be classified as
a. Bench-top or floor model
b. With refrigeration and without refrigeration
c. Based on rotor design
d. Based on maximum speed which can be attained (normal or ultracentrifuge)

Q5. What is the rotor in a centrifuge?
Ans. Rotor is the component of the centrifuge machine which is holding the tubes or vacutainers. Based on rotor design, we have two types of centrifuge:
- Horizontal rotor type (swing out head)
- Fixed angle rotor type (angle head)

Q6. What is the principle of centrifuge?
Ans. Principle of centrifuge machine
Key factor in separating the particulate matter from liquid suspension is the relative centrifugal force (RCF) which is represented by following formula

$$RCF = R \times (RPM)^2 \times 118 \times 10^{-7}$$

R is the rotating radius of the rotor which means the radius of rotating path from the central axis.
RPM (revolution per minute): It is the number of revolution of rotor in a minute. It can be programmed in the centrifuge.

Q7. What is ultracentrifuge? Mention its use.
Ans. The centrifuge which can be operated at very high speed (1,00,000 RPM) is known as ultracentrifuge.
This is used for:
1. Drying of the glassware
2. Heating the chemicals wherever required
3. Dry sterilization of glassware (in microbiological experiments mainly), metal equipment, swabs, etc. (in surgical units).

Q8. What is desiccator and what is desiccant?
Ans. Desiccator and desiccants
Desiccants are hygroscopic substances which absorb water from atmosphere and from various other hydrated substances. In other words, desiccants are drying agents.
In biochemical lab, we need to remove moisture from many chemicals before using them for analytical purpose, for that these chemicals are kept in contact with desiccants in a closed, airtight chamber with a lid with a lubricated seal is known as desiccator.

Q9. What is pH?
Ans. pH of a solution is negative logarithm of the hydrogen ion concentration. It can be expressed as

$$pH = 1/\log 10\,(H^+)$$

As stated in equation above, pH of a solution is inversely proportional to its hydrogen ion concentration.

Plasma = 7.35 to 7.45 [Mean = 7.4]
Urine = 6.5
CSF = 7.32
Gastric juice = 1.0 to 2.0

Q10. Mention the difference between Mohr pipette and serological pipette.
Ans.
Mohr type: Mohr pipette does not have graduations till tip and it is self-draining type.
Serological type: Serological pipette has graduation till tip and is blowout type.

Notes

CHAPTER 2

Safe Laboratory Practice and Waste Disposal

> **Competency**
>
> **BI 11.1:** Describe good safe laboratory practice and waste disposal.

LABORATORY SAFETY

All clinical laboratory personnel are constantly exposed to various hazards like electric shock, radioactive material hazard, gaseous hazard, corrosive substances, and risk of handling biological material.

Recognition of hazard in the lab is of foremost importance along with the right attitude of the employer and employee towards safety measures to have a safe lab practice.

Safety Awareness for Laboratory Personnel

- Both employer and employee need to share the responsibility for effective implementation of safety practices in the lab.
- Employer need to formulate the laboratory work methods and safety policies and should provide time-to-time training to all employees.
- Personal protective equipment (PPE) consisting of gloves, eye shield, apron, cap, shoe cover should be provided to them. Employee should comply with the guidelines and should have positive attitude towards safety practices.
- Signage and labelling should be used liberally to identify the critical hazards and guidelines for precautions should be displayed at appropriate places.

Biological Safety

Clinical lab personnel deal with potential infectious blood and other biological samples. Utmost care should be taken while collecting, transporting, processing and analyzing such samples. Proper gloves, gowns, face protection should be practiced while handling such samples.

Any infectious material (blood, urine, or any other biological material), if spilled, should be taken care. 10% bleach should be used at spill site for appropriate time and then the site should be rinsed with water.

All the blood and other biological samples should be handled taking universal precaution considering all of them as potentially infectious.

Chemical Safety

Material safety data sheets (MSDS) for each hazardous compound at workplace should be obtained and all employees should be educated for its use and they should be clearly explained how to work safely with the chemicals.

Fire Safety

Fire extinguisher should be placed at appropriate place and all lab personnel should be trained for its use at the time of need.

Radiation Safety

All the places where radioactive material is stored should be labelled with cautious signage and entry of only authorized personnel should be allowed.

Disposal of Hazardous Material

Chemical material disposal: Most of the water-soluble chemicals may be flushed in the drain with large amount of water. Strong acid and strong bases should be neutralized first before discarding them in drain.

Possible chemical reaction in the drain between certain chemicals should be kept in mind and due precaution is to be taken. Foul smelling chemicals should not be disposed directly, rather they should be diluted first before being dumped in the drain.

Solid chemical waste can be buried in a landfill.

Radioactive material disposal: Radioactive material should be handed over to licensed receiver for safe disposal.

Handling Accidental Exposure to Acid and Alkali

Exposure to Acid

Various acids used in biochemistry laboratory are: Hydrochloric acid, nitric acid, sulfuric acid and acetic acid.

Exposure to skin

1. Wash with large quantity of water.
2. Apply 5% sodium carbonate solution with cotton wool.

Exposure to eye

1. Spray large quantity of water in eye.
2. Add 3 to 4 drops of 2% sodium carbonate in eye every 5 minutes till you consult ophthalmologist.

Swallowing of acid

1. Ask patient to drink 2 white of egg mixed in water or milk, alternatively ask him to drink soap water.
2. Ask him to gargle with soap water as well.
3. Ask him to drink 500 mL of normal water as well.
4. Apply 2% sodium bicarbonate to lips and tongue, if they are also burnt.

Exposure to Alkali

Commonly used alkalis in biochemistry laboratory are: Sodium hydroxide, ammonium hydroxide, and potassium hydroxide.

Exposure to skin
1. Wash with large quantity of water.
2. Apply 5% acetic acid with cotton wool.

Exposure to eye
1. Spray large quantity of water in eye.
2. Add 3 to 4 drops of saturated boric acid in eye every 5 minutes till you consult ophthalmologist.

Swallowing of alkali
1. Ask patient to drink lemon juice or diluted vinegar (1:3/vinegar: water).
2. Ask him to gargle with same acid solution.
3. Ask him to drink 500 mL of normal water as well.
4. Apply 5% acetic acid solution to lips and tongue, if they are also burnt.

BIOMEDICAL WASTE (BMW) MANAGEMENT

Difference between Hospital Waste and Biomedical Waste

Hospital waste: It refers to all waste, biological or non-biological that is discarded and not intended for further use.

Biomedical waste: It is defined as **"any solid, fluid and liquid or liquid waste, including its container and any intermediate product, which is generated during the diagnosis, treatment or immunization of human being or animals".**

According to WHO:
- Nearly 85% of all waste generated by hospital is general waste.
- About 15% waste is biomedical waste, which includes:
  - Infectious waste—10%.
  - Non-infectious waste such as radioactive and chemical wastes—5%.

Why there is a Need of BMW Management?

Hospitals generate substantial quantity of waste that has potential to cause health and environmental hazards. Safe and sustainable management of biomedical waste (BMW) is social and legal responsibility of all people supporting and financing healthcare activities.

The need for effective biomedical waste management is due to following risks:
1. **Risk of infection** outside hospital for waste handlers, scavengers and at times, general public living in the vicinity of the hospitals.
2. **Injuries from sharps** leading to infection to all categories of hospital personnel and waste handlers.
3. **Risk associated with hazardous chemicals** and drugs to persons handling wastes at all levels.
4. Nosocomial infections in patients from poor infection control practices and poor waste management.
5. **Risk of recycling of "disposables"** which are being repacked and sold.
6. Risk of air, water and soil pollution directly due to waste, or due to defective incineration, emissions and ash.

On March 28, 2016, the Government of India published the **"Biomedical Waste Management Rules, 2016"** in supersession of the Biomedical Waste (Management and Handling) Rules, 1998.

Salient Features of BMW Management Rules, 2016 along with Bio-Medical Waste Management (Amendment) Rules, 2018

1. The scope of the rules has been expanded to include vaccination camps, blood donation camps, surgical camps or any other healthcare activity.
2. Phase-out the use of chlorinated plastic bags, gloves and blood bags within two years of notification of BMW Management 2016 Rules, i.e. by 27th March, 2018.
3. But as per the Bio-Medical Waste Management (Amendment) Rules, 2018, use of chlorinated plastic bags (excluding blood bags) and gloves has to be phased out by the 27th March, 2019.
4. Pre-treatment of the laboratory waste, microbiological waste, blood samples and blood bags through disinfection sterilization on-site in the manner as prescribed by WHO or NACO.
5. Provide training to all its healthcare workers and immunize all health workers regularly against diseases like tetanus and hepatitis B.
6. Establish a Bar-Code System for bags or containers containing biomedical waste for disposal within one year of notification of rules, i.e. 27th March, 2017. But as per the Bio-Medical Waste Management (Amendment) Rules, 2018, Bar-Code System has to be established in accordance with the guidelines issued by the Central Pollution Control Board by 27th March, 2019.
7. Report major accidents like needle stick injuries, broken mercury thermometer, accidents caused by fire, blasts during handling of biomedical waste and the remedial action taken.
8. Procedure to get authorization is simplified.
9. The new rules prescribe more stringent standards for incinerator to reduce the emission of pollutants in environment.
10. No hospital/healthcare facility (occupier) shall establish on-site treatment and disposal facility, if a service of "common biomedical waste treatment facility" (CBMWTF) is available at 75 km.
11. Operator of a common biomedical waste treatment and disposal facility to ensure the timely collection of biomedical waste from the healthcare facility and assist the healthcare facility in conducting training.

Steps in the management of biomedical waste include:
a. Generation
b. Segregation
c. Collection
d. Storage
e. Treatment
f. Transport
g. Disposal.

Colour Coding of Biomedical Wastes and their Disposal

Bio-Medical Waste Management Rules, 2016 has categorized the biomedical waste generated from the healthcare facility into four categories based on the segregation pathway and colour code.

Various types of biomedical waste are further assigned to each one of the categories, as detailed below **(Fig. 2.1):**

1. Yellow category
2. Red category

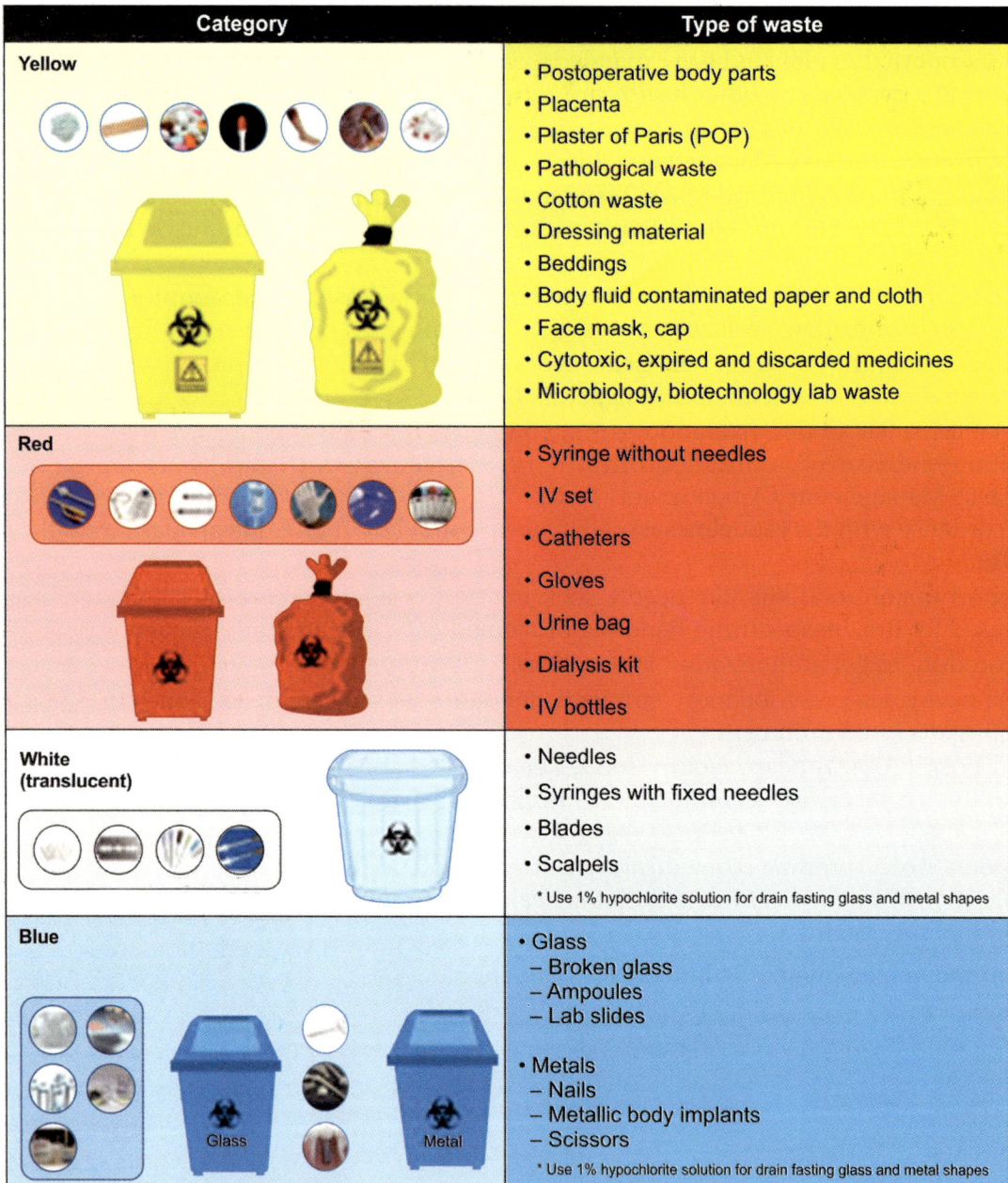

Fig. 2.1: Color coding of biowaste container

    3. White category
    4. Black category

Biomedical wastes' categories and their segregation, collection, treatment, processing and disposal options are summarized in Table 2.1.

Table 2.1: Biomedical wastes' categories and their processing

Category	Type of waste	Type of bag or container to be used	Treatment and disposal options
Yellow	a. **Human anatomical waste**	Yellow-coloured non-chlorinated plastic bags	Incineration or plasma pyrolysis or deep burial
	b. **Animal anatomical waste**		
	c. **Chemical liquid waste:** Liquid waste generated due to use of chemicals in production of biological and used or discarded disinfectants, silver X-ray film developing liquid, discarded formalin, infected secretions, aspirated body fluids		
	d. **Soiled waste:** Items contaminated with blood, body fluids like dressings, plaster casts, cotton swabs and bags containing residual or discarded blood and blood components		Incineration or plasma pyrolysis or deep burial* In absence of above facilities, autoclaving or microwaving/ hydroclaving followed by shredding or mutilation or combination of sterilization and shredding.
	e. **Expired or discarded medicines:** Pharmaceutical waste like antibiotics, cytotoxic drugs including all items contaminated with cytotoxic drugs along with glass or plastic ampoules, vials, etc.	Yellow-coloured non-chlorinated plastic bags or containers	Expired cytotoxic drugs and items contaminated with cytotoxic drugs to be returned back to the manufacturer or supplier for incineration at temperature >1200°C
	f. **Discarded linen, mattresses, beddings contaminated with blood or body fluid**	Non-chlorinated yellow plastic bags or suitable packing material	Non-chlorinated chemical disinfection followed by incineration or plazma pyrolysis or for energy recovery. In absence of above facilities, shredding or mutilation or combination of sterilization and shredding.
	g. **Microbiology, biotechnology and other clinical laboratory waste:** Blood bags, laboratory cultures, stocks or specimens of microorganisms, live or attenuated vaccines, human and animal cell cultures used in research, industrial laboratories	Autoclave safe plastic bags or containers	Pre-treat to sterilize with non-chlorinated chemicals on-site as per National AIDS Control Organization or World Health Organization guidelines thereafter for incineration

(Contd.)

Table 2.1: Biomedical wastes' categories and their processing (Contd.)			
Category	Type of waste	Type of bag or container to be used	Treatment and disposal options
Red	**Contaminated waste (recyclable):** Wastes such as tubing, bottles, intravenous tubes and sets, catheters, urine bags, syringes (without needles and *fixed needle syringes*), vacutainers, gloves	Red-coloured non-chlorinated plastic bags or containers	Autoclaving or microwaving/hydroclaving followed by shredding or mutilation or combination of sterilization and shredding. Treated material can be recycled
White (translucent)	**Waste sharps including metals:** Needles, syringes with fixed needles, needles from needle tip cutter or burner, scalpels, blades, or any other contaminated sharp object that may cause puncture and cuts	Puncture-proof, leak-proof, tamper-proof containers	Autoclaving or dry heat sterilization followed by shredding or mutilation or encapsulation in metal container. Combination of shredding cum autoclaving; and sent for final disposal to iron foundries
Blue	a. **Glassware:** Broken or discarded and contaminated glass including medicine vials and ampoules (except those contaminated with cytotoxic wastes) b. **Metallic body implants**	Cardboard boxes with blue-coloured marking Cardboard boxes with blue-coloured marking	Disinfection (by soaking in sodium hypochlorite) or through autoclaving or microwaving or hydroclaving and then sent for recycling

Safe Laboratory Practice and Waste Disposal

VIVA VOCE

Q1. How will you handle the acid spill on hand of your colleague?

Ans. *Exposure to skin*

1. Wash with large quantity of water.
2. Apply 5% sodium carbonate solution with cotton wool.

Q2. What is to be done in case of accidental ingestion of acid?

Ans. *Swallowing of acid*

1. Ask patient to drink 2 white of egg mixed in water or milk, alternatively ask him to drink soap water.
2. Ask him to gargle with soap water as well.
3. Ask him to drink 500 ml of normal water as well.
4. Apply 2% sodium bicarbonate to lips and tongue, if they are also burnt.

Q3. How will you handle the alkali spill on hand of your colleague?

Ans. *Exposure to skin*

1. Wash with large quantity of water.
2. Apply 5% acetic acid with cotton wool.

Q4. What is to be done in case of accidental ingestion of alkali?

Ans. *Swallowing of alkali*

1. Ask patient to drink lemon juice or diluted vinegar (1:3/vinegar:water).
2. Ask him to gargle with same acid solution.
3. Ask him to drink 500 ml of normal water as well.
4. Apply 5% acetic acid solution to lips and tongue, if they are also burnt.

Q5. What is biomedical waste?

Ans. *Biomedical waste* is defined as "any solid, fluid and liquid or liquid waste, including its container and any intermediate product, which is generated during the diagnosis, treatment or immunization of human being or animals".

Q6. What is the need of effective biomedical waste management?

Ans. The need for effective biomedical waste management is due to following risks:

1. Risk of infection outside hospital for waste handlers and scavengers and at times, general public living in the vicinity of the hospitals.
2. Injuries from sharps leading to infection to all categories of hospital personnel and waste handlers.
3. Risk associated with hazardous chemicals and drugs to persons handling wastes at all levels.
4. Nosocomial infections in patients from poor infection control practices and poor waste management.
5. Risk of recycling of "disposables" which are being repacked and sold.
6. Risk of air, water and soil pollution directly due to waste, or due to defective incineration, emissions and ash.

Q7. How to discard broken glass ampoules?

Ans. Broken or discarded and contaminated glass including medicine vials and ampoules (except those contaminated with cytotoxic wastes.)

Notes

Section II

Qualitative Assessments

3. Analysis of Normal Urine for Its Constituents
4. Analysis of Abnormal Constituents in the Urine and Their Clinical Correlation

CHAPTER

3

Analysis of Normal Urine for Its Constituents

> **Competencies**
>
> **BI 11.3:** Describe the chemical components of normal urine.
> **BI 11.4:** Perform urine analysis to estimate and determine normal compounds in the urine.
> **PE 21.11:** Perform and interpret the common constituent analyte in a urine examination.

This chapter deals with discussion on normal urine. For discussion on abnormal urine, kindly refer the Chapter 4.

FORMATION OF URINE

Urine is formed in both the kidneys. It is the ultrafiltrate of plasma which is produced when blood passes through both the glomeruli. Formation of urine is an important measure by which body gets rid of excretory substances. Out of total 180 L of glomerular filtrate each day, only 1.5 L of urine is finally formed after extensive reabsorption of glomerular filtrate by the tubules and also by secretion of water and solutes in the tubular lumen.

Normal urine is pale strawcolor, transparent fluid which is having ammoniacal smell.

Why Evaluation of Urine is Important?

Evaluation of urine helps determining the functioning of kidney (glomerulus and tubules) and is also useful in diagnosis and severity of many other diseases like, diabetes mellitus, nephrotic syndrome, jaundice, nephropathy, metabolic diseases like various aminoacidurias.

Collection of Urine

Collection of 24-hour urine: 24-hour urine collection is needed for estimation of total urine output in a day and also for assessment of total protein and calcium in urine.

For such collection, preservatives need to be used. 10 mL of conc. HCl can be poured in jar meant to collect 24-hour urine. Patient is advised to collect all the urine of 24 hours after discarding the first morning urine.

Morning mid-stream sample collection: For collection of morning mid-stream sample, patient is advised to discard initial 5–10 mL of urine and next 10–15 mL of urine is collected for routine analysis.

Random urine collection: Random urine is the urine collected at any time of the day. This urine is adequate for estimation of most of the analyte in the urine.

Following are the physical characteristics of fresh 'normal urine' in a healthy adult:
1. Appearance   : Clear, transparent
2. Volume   : 1.5 to 2.5 L [1500 to 2500 mL] in a day
3. Color   : Amber yellow (pale yellow/straw colored)
4. Odor   : Ammoniacal odor
5. pH   : Acidic pH is 6.5 [turns blue litmus to red]
6. Specific gravity : 1.010 to 1.020

These characteristics are being discussed one by one.

Appearance

Urine may be turbid or cloudy due to presence of any of the following:
- Pus
- Bacteria
- Fungi
- Chyluria (lipid in urine)

In addition, presence of phosphate and urate also imparts cloudiness to urine.

Volume

Normal volume of 24-hour urine in a healthy adult on normal fluid intake is 1500 to 2500 mL.

Conditions of excess passage of urine is polyuria and the conditions where lesser or nil urine is passed in 24-hour is known as oliguria or anuria, respectively.

Abnormal volume of urine and disease conditions associated with it		
Polyuria:	>2500 mL	Diabetes mellitus, diabetes insipidus, excess fluid intake, diuretics
Oliguria:	<300 mL	Low BP, shock, acute tubular neurosis, prostate enlargement
Anuria:	Nil urine in 24-hour	Seen in tumor and calculi

Color

Normal urine has pale yellow color which is due to excretion of urobilinogen. Urine color changes in certain diseases which helps in diagnosis. For example:
- *Yellow color*: Jaundice
- *Black color*: Alkaptonuria
- *Red color*: Hematuria, rifampicin intake, excess beet root consumption.

Odor

Fresh urine has aromatic smell, but urine on standing for few hours develop ammoniacal odor due to decomposition of urea.

Fruity odor of urine denotes possibility of ketone body (acetone) in the urine. In addition, in many "aminoacidurias", urine gives characteristic odor due to excretion of metabolic intermediates.

For example, here is the list of certain important odors which are very helpful in diagnosis.

Odor	Disorder
Mousy or musty	Phenylketonuria
Cheesy	Isovaleric aciduria
Burnt sugar	Branched chain ketonuria (MSUD)
Cabbage	Tyrosinosis (tyrosinemia type I)

pH
- Normal urine pH ranges from 4.8 to 7.8 and it varies widely with diet.
- Urine on standing turns alkaline due to decomposition of urea which produces ammonia.
- Extreme of pH denotes faulty urine collection.
- pH of urine may be assessed by pH paper or dipsticks.

Specific Gravity

Specific gravity of the urine is a **crude measure of total solute excreted in the urine**. Normal specific gravity of the urine varies from 1.010 to 1.020.

1. *Conditions where specific gravity is decreased*:
   - Diabetes insipidus
   - Polyuria
   - Excess water intake
   - Diuretics intake
2. *Conditions where specific gravity is increased*:
   - Diabetes mellitus
   - Proteinuria
   - Dehydration
   - Less water intake [hence passing of concentrated urine]

Measurement of Specific Gravity

Specific gravity of urine can be measured by an instrument known as **"Urinometer"** (Fig. 3.1).

Urinometer is a glass instrument which has a bulb and a stem. Bulb is filled with mercury and stem is having marks ranging from 1.000 to 1.060 (Fig. 3.2).

This instrument is calibrated at 15°C and hence temperature correction is done based on at what room temperature the measurement is being done.

For every 3°C of temperature beyond 15°C, 0.001 is added in measured value and for every 3°C temperature below 15°C, 0.001 is deducted from measured value.

> For example,
> If the room temperature, where the measurement is being done is 24°C, then: 3 × 0.001 = 0.003 should be added in the measured value.
> Room temperature = 24°C
> Temperature of calibration = 15°C
> Difference is plus 9°C
> For every 3°C rise of T°, correction factor is 0.001 so for 9°C rise correction factor is +0.003.

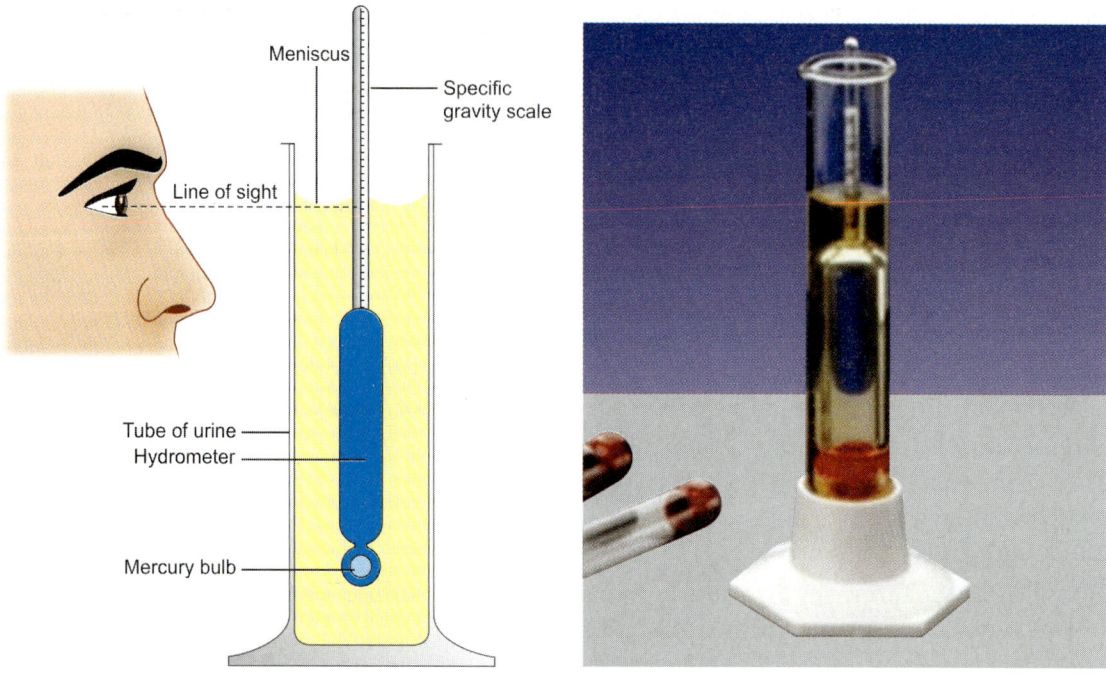

Fig. 3.1: Urinometer

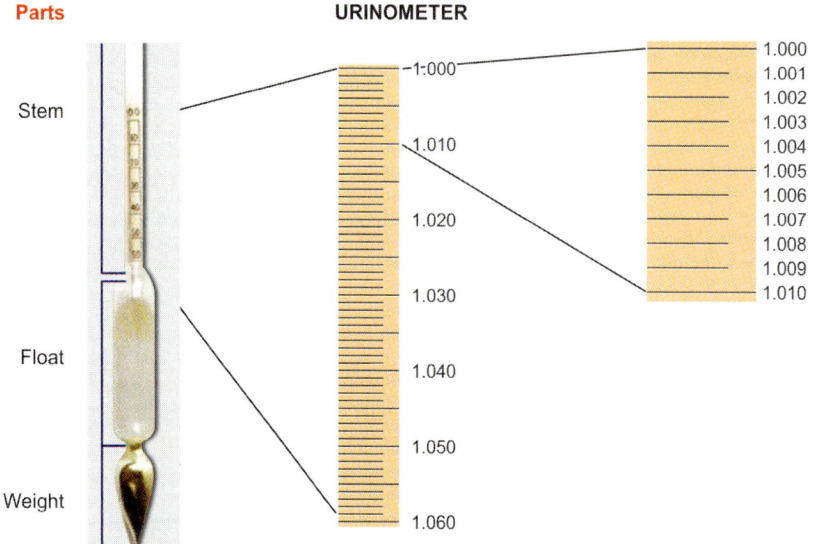

Fig. 3.2: Marking on stem of urinometer

Similarly, suppose if the measurement is done at room T° of 12°C, then 0.001 need to be deducted from measured value of specific gravity.

Room temperature = 12°C
T° of calibration = 15°C
Difference is minus 3°C
For every 3°C decline in T° below 15°C, the factor to be deducted is 0.001.

Normal urine contains both organic and inorganic constituents. Following are organic and inorganic constituents of the urine.

Organic Constituents
- *Urea*: It is the chief nitrogenous component of the urine. Urea is the end product of protein metabolism.
- *Uric acid*: It is the end product of purine nucleotide metabolism.
- *Creatinine*: It is excretory compound produced by spontaneous dehydration of creatine.
- *Urobilinogen*: It is produced after degradation of bilirubin in the intestinal lumen and enters in enterohepatic circulation.

Inorganic Constituents
- Sodium (Na^+)
- Potassium (K^+)
- Calcium (Ca^{++})
- Magnesium (Mg^{++})
- Ammonium (NH_4^+)
- Chloride (Cl^-)
- Phosphate (PO_4^{3-})
- Sulphate (SO_4^{2-})
- Bicarbonate (HCO_3^-)

Tests for Organic Constituents of Normal Urine
Tables 3.1 to 3.4 depict the tests for organic constituents of normal urine.

Table 3.1: Test for urea		
Experiments	*Observation*	*Inference*
Alkaline hypobromite test 3 mL of urine + few drops of alkaline hypobromite	Brisk effervescence is seen coming out of the test tube Effervescence	Urea is present in urine N_2 of urea emitted as brisk effervescence $NH_2CONH_2 + 3NaOBr$ $\downarrow$ Emitted as an effervescence I. $3NaBr + \boxed{N_2} + CO_2 + 2H$ II. $CO_2 + NaOH\,(2) \rightarrow Na_2CO_3 + 2H_2O$
Specific urease test 2 mL urine + two drops of phenol red*+ drops of acetic acid (2%) till pink color disappears. Then add 1 mL of urease enzyme	Solution turns pink	Urea is present in urine Urea present is acted upon by urease enzyme to produce ammonium carbonate which turns solution pink due to phenol red

*Phenol red turn red in alkaline medium.

Table: 3.2: Test for uric acid

Experiment	Observation	Inference
Shiff's test A strip of filter paper is moistened with 3% ammoniacal $AgNO_3$ + few drops of uric acid added	Filter paper turns black	Uric acid present This is due to reduction of $AgNO_3$ to free silver in alkaline medium
Benedict's uric acid test 5 mL of urine + 1–2 g of anhydrous Na_2CO_3 + 5–6 drops of Benedict's uric acid reagent	Intense blue color observed	Uric acid converts phosphotungstic acid to tungsten blue in alkaline medium

Murexide test for uric acid (used in stone analysis)
Pinch of uric acid in petridish + 2–3 drops of conc. HNO_3 + heat it on water bath till it dries.
Divide in two parts:
Part I: Add drops of $(NH_4)_2OH$ → Purplish red
Part II: Add drops of KOH → Purplish violet

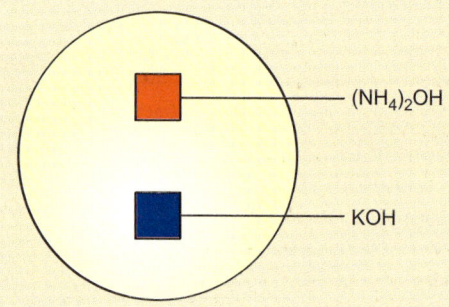

Table 3.3: Test for creatinine

Experiment	Observation	Inference
Jaffe's test Take 5 mL of saturated picric acid in a test tube + 5 mL of 5% NaOH Total 10 mL Divide it into 2 test tubes (5 mL each)		

(Contd.)

Table 3.3: Test for creatinine (Contd.)

Experiment	Observation	Inference
TT (1): Add 5 mL of DW [control tube]	No change in color	Creatinine present in urine
TT (2): Add 5 mL of urine solution and mix [test]	Orange red color	Creatinine reacts with alkaline picrate to produce creatinine picrate which gives orange red color

Table 3.4: Test for urobilinogen (UBG)

Experiment	Observation	Inference
Ehrlich's test 5 mL of urine + 1 mL of Ehrlich reagent. Keep it for 5 min at room temperature Observe the color change and compare with unprocessed urine	Red color	Presence of urobilinogen in the urine. UBG reacts with p-dimethyl amino-benzaldehyde to give red-colored complex

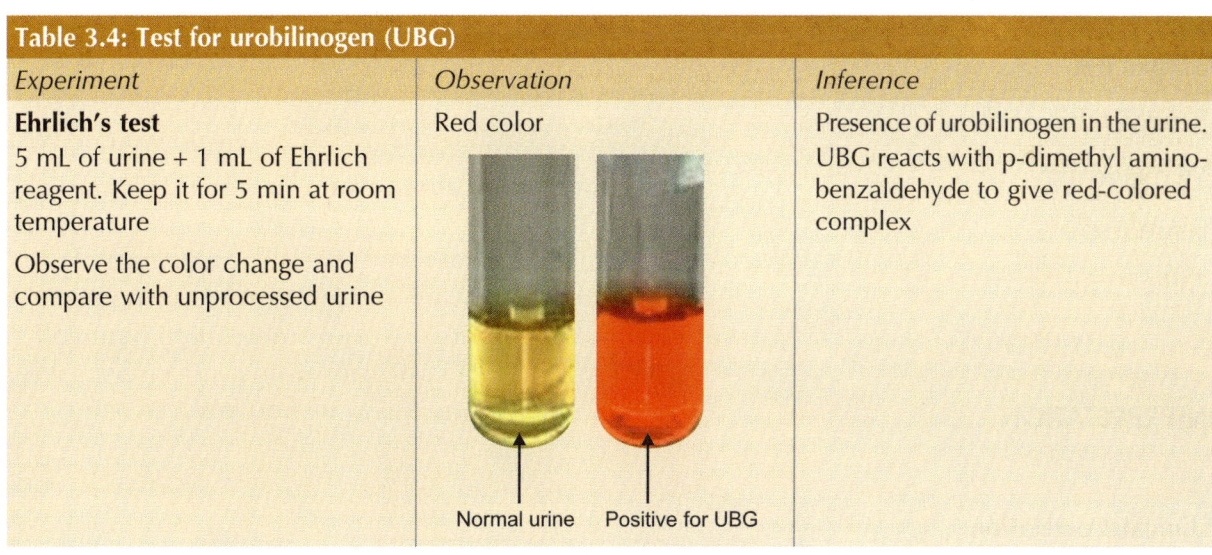

Normal urine   Positive for UBG

Experiment Name: Examination of urine for normal constituents

OBSERVATION

Physical Characteristics

Appearance: _____

Volume: _____

Color: _____

Odor: _____

pH: _____

Specific gravity: _____

Analysis of Normal Constituents

Experiment	Observation	Inference
Alkaline hypobromite test		
Specific urease test		
Schiff's test		
Benedict uric acid test		
Murexide test		
Jaffe's test		
Ehrlich's test		

INTERPRETATION

Clinical Correlation: _____

_____

_____

_____

Dated: _____   **Teacher's Signature**

Analysis of Normal Urine for Its Constituents

VIVA VOCE

Q1. Why there is need of collection of 24-hour urine?
Ans. 24-hour urine collection is needed for estimation of total urine output in a day and also for assessment of total protein and calcium in urine.

Q2. What all precautions will be taken while advising 24-hour collection of urine?
Ans. For such collection, preservatives need to be used. 10 mL of conc. HCl can be poured in jar meant to collect 24-hour urine. Patient is advised to collect all the urine of 24 hours after discarding the first morning urine.

Q3. What is the normal pH of the urine?
Ans. Normal pH of urine is acidic. [pH is 6.5—turns blue litmus to red]

Q4. What is polyuria?
Ans. If 24-hour urine volume is >2500 mL, the condition is called polyuria.
  It is seen in following conditions:
  - Diabetes mellitus
  - Diabetes insipidus
  - Excess fluid intake
  - Diuretics

Q5. What is oliguria?
Ans. If 24-hour urine collection is <300 mL, it is called oliguria.
  It is seen in following conditions:
  - Low BP
  - Shock
  - Acute tubular neurosis
  - Prostate enlargement

Q6. Enumerate certain conditions when red urine is passed.
Ans. Red urine is observed in following conditions:
- Hematuria (blood in urine due to injury of malignancy of urinary tract)
- Rifampicin intake
- Excess beetroot consumption

Q7. What is the normal specific gravity of urine?
Ans. Normal specific gravity of the urine varies from 1.010 to 1.020.

Q8. How the correction of temperature is done while estimating the specif gravity of urine using urinometer?
Ans. Urinometer instrument is calibrated at 15°C and hence temperature correction is done based on at what room temperature the measurement is being done.
- For every 3°C of temperature beyond 15°C, 0.001 is added in measured value and for every 3°C temperature below 15°C, 0.001 is deducted from measured value.

CHAPTER

4

Analysis of Abnormal Constituents in the Urine and Their Clinical Correlation

> **Competencies**
>
> **BI 11.4:** Perform urine analysis to estimate and determine abnormal constituents.
> **BI 11.20:** Identify abnormal constituents in urine, interpret the findings and correlate these with pathological states.
> **IM11.13/Vertical integration:** Perform and interpret a urinary ketone estimation with a dipstick.
> **PE33.6/Vertical integration:** Perform and interpret urine dipstick for sugar.

In this segment, students will learn about various abnormal constituents of urine and methods for detecting them in patient's urine.

Following abnormal constituents may be found in the urine depending upon the disease status:
1. Reducing sugar
2. Proteins
3. Bile pigments
4. Bile salt
5. Ketone body
6. Blood

REDUCING SUGARS

Reducing sugars which come out in the urine and corresponding diseases are represented in Table 4.1.

Table 4.1: Various reducing sugars and diseases in which they are excreted in urine		
Reducing sugar	*Disease in which it may be excreted in urine*	*Remarks*
Glucose	Diabetes mellitus	Renal threshold for glucose is 180 mg/dL, beyond which glucose comes out in the urine
Galactose	Galactosemia	Disorder of galactose metabolism
Fructose	Essential fructosuria and hereditary fructose intolerance	Disorder of fructose metabolism
L-xylulose	Essential pentosuria	Disorder of uronic acid and pathway
Lactose	Pregnancy	

Out of various reducing sugars enumerated in Table 4.1, excretion of glucose in the urine is the commonest finding as the corresponding disease [diabetes mellitus] is most prevalent.

Most commonly used test for detection of reducing sugar in the urine is **'Benedict's test'** which is based on reducing property of these sugars. Reducing sugar reduces cupric ion (Cu^{++}) of copper sulfate to cuprous ion (Cu^+) which forms cuprous oxide (Cu_2O) which gives different shades of color based on the quantity of cuprous oxide.

This test is **'semiquantitative test'** because the color, which is developed, gives the appropriate value of reducing sugar in the urine.

For doing this test, 5 mL of Benedict's solution is taken in the test tube and eight drops of urine is added in it. After mixing it thoroughly, bottom of test tube is heated or kept in a boiling water bath for 2 min. Color developed on cooling is noted and interpreted (Table 4.2).

Ratio of Benedict's solution and urine should be maintained as 5 mL of Benedict's solution: 8 drops of urine (or 2.5 mL: 4 drops) while doing the test as the test is semiquantitative and color developed in the test tube depends upon the amount of reducing sugars in the urine.

In addition to reducing sugars, certain non-carbohydrate substances also give this test positive. These substances are:
- Vitamin C (ascorbic acid)
- Homogentisic acid (HGA)
- Creatinine
- Uric acid
- Salicylates

Condition when glucose comes out in the urine is called glucosuria.

Detection of Glucose in Urine by Dipstick Method

[*Compentency PE 33.6*]

Stiff cellulose strips which are coated with 'glucose oxidase' is sensitive and specific method for detection of glucose in the urine. On dipping the strip in urine, if strips turn purple, it detects the presence of glucose in the urine. This test may detect even small amount of glucose in the urine (<0.1 g%) (hence sensitive).

This test is based on principle of GOD-POD (glucose oxidase-peroxidase). (Hence, it is specific for glucose detection—Table 4.3 and Fig. 4.1.)

$$\text{Glucose} \xrightarrow{GOD} \text{Gluconic acid} + H_2O_2$$

$$H_2O_2 \xrightarrow{POD} H_2O + [O]$$

$$\text{Orthotoluidine} + [O] \longrightarrow \text{Colored complex}$$

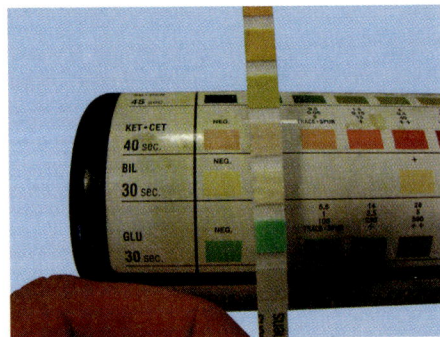

Fig. 4.1: Detection of glucose in urine by 'dipstick method'

Analysis of Abnormal Constituents in the Urine and Their Clinical Correlation

Table 4.2: Color developed and quantity of reducing sugar in the urine

Color/precipitate observed	Illustration	Quantity of sugar in urine (g%)
Blue color		Absence of sugar
Green color		<0.5 g%
Green precipitate		0.5 to 1.0 g% (+)
Yellow precipitate		>1.0–1.5 g% (++)
Orange precipitate		>1.5 to 2 g% (+++)
Red precipitate		>2 g% (++++)

Table 4.3: Detection of glucose in urine by 'dipstick method'		
Procedure	Observation	Inference
Take 5 mL of urine in test tube		
Dip one end of strip in the urine	No change of color	No glucose in urine
Read the color after 30 sec	Color change to purple	Glucose in urine is positive

PROTEINS

Protein in urine is called proteinuria. Predominant protein which is lost in urine during proteinuria is albumin which is filtered because of its small size.

Condition which damages the basement membrane (nephropathy) results in proteinuria.

There are many methods which can detect the presence of protein in the urine, and all these methods are based on precipitation of protein. These methods are:

1. Heat coagulation test
2. Heller's test
3. Sulfosalicylic acid test
4. Salting out
5. Precipitation with the help of volatile solvents (alcohol/acetone)
6. Isoelectric pH (pI)

To understand the principle of various methods used for protein precipitation, it is first of all important to understand the reason for protein solubility.

There are three factors which are important for protein solubility:

 i. Intact tertiary structure of protein
 ii. Net change on the particle
 iii. Shell of hydration around it

If either the protein is denatured or shell of hydration is disrupted with or without nullification of charge, protein gets precipitated.

Methods of Denaturation of Protein and Its Precipitation

Denaturation is a phenomenon where protein loses its quaternary, tertiary, and secondary structures; while primary structure is maintained.

Protein can be denatured by using heat, strong acid, strong alkali, urea, radiation, etc.

Method 1, 2, 3 enumerated above are based on protein denaturation.

Denaturation of Protein Using Heat (Heat Coagulation Test)

This is commonly used method to detect the protein in the urine (Table 4.4).

Albustix for Detection of Albumin (Fig. 4.2)

This test is based on principle that protein alter the color of certain acid-base indicator, such as TBP blue (tetrabromophenol blue). When the dye is buffered at pH 3, it is yellow. Protein changes this color to green to blue depending upon its concentration. Comparison of developed color with color chart helps in grading the concentration of protein from traces to +4 (1–10 to >500 mg/dL).

Precipitation of Protein Using Strong Acid (Conc. HNO_3) (Heller's Test)

Conc. HNO_3 is a strong denaturant. It tends to denature the protein once it comes in contact with it (Table 4.5).

Analysis of Abnormal Constituents in the Urine and Their Clinical Correlation

Table 4.4: Heat coagulation test

Procedure	Observation	Inference
Fill ¾ of the test tube with the urine and heat upper one-third of its by putting the upper 1/3rd of TT over the slow flame. Heat for a min. Lower 2/3rd of urine in TT serves as a control	White turbidity appears on heating and **gets dissolved** after addition of 1% acetic acid	The white ppt was because of phosphate or carbonate which got dissolved by acetic acid
	White turbidity appears on heating which **gets intensified** on addition of 1% acetic acid	White ppt was because of protein (albumin). Addition of 1% acetic acid bought the pH of urine nearer to pI of albumin and intensified the precipitate.

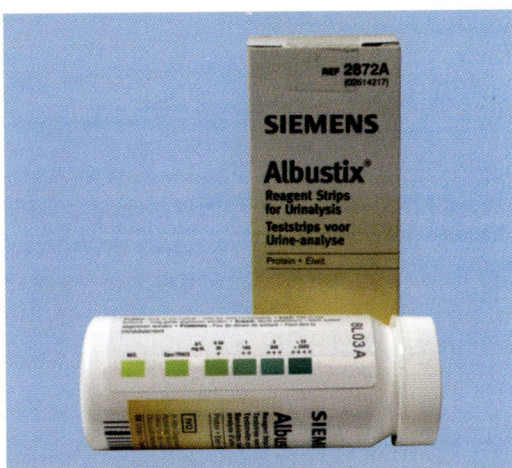

Fig. 4.2: Albustix test

Table 4.5: Heller's test

Procedure	Observation	Inference
5 mL of urine is taken in a test tube. 1 mL of conc. HNO_3 is added in the urine drop by drop from the side of the test tube	A white ring appears at the junction of two liquids which denotes denatured protein	Presence of protein in the urine

Precipitation of Protein Using Sulfosalicylic Acid

After centrifuging the urine, 2.5 mL of supernatant is added to 7.5 mL of 3% sulfosalicylic acid. Degree of turbidity is quantified as given in Table 4.6.

Table 4.6: Interpretation of sulfosalicylic acid test for protein precipitation

Protein (mg/dL)	Degree of turbidity
0	Clear
1–10	Opalescent
15–30	Can read print through tube
40–100	Can read only black line
150–400	No visible black lines
>500	Flocculent

Methods of Denaturation of Protein by Disruption of Shell of Hydration with or without Charge Nullification

Shell of hydration may be disrupted by following:
 i. Salting out
 ii. Alcohol/acetone (volatile solvent)

Salting Out

For it, most preferred salt used is ammonium sulfate which is highly soluble in polar medium (H_2O/urine). Hence, when excess of $(NH_4)_2SO_4$ is dissolved in urine, in an attempt to solubilize itself, it drags the shell of hydration from the proteins and hence proteins are precipitated.

Albumin gets precipitated with full saturation and globulin tends to get precipitate with half saturation.

(Albumin being smaller in size than globulin, has got more surface area hence needs full saturation with ammonium sulfate salt and globulin being large in size has got lesser surface area and hence gets precipitated in half saturation with salt.)

Using Alcohol and Acetone

Alcohol and acetone are volatile solvents and they tend to evaporate the shell of hydration from around the protein, when a few drops of these solvents are added in the solution containing protein and is vigorously shaken (Table 4.7).

Table 4.7: Precipitation of protein by alcohol or acetone

Procedure	Observation	Inference
Take 3 mL urine in a test tube + add 4 drops of alcohol or acetone + shake it vigorously	White ppt seen No ppt is seen	Protein is present in urine Protein is absent in urine

Bringing the pH to Isoelectric pH (pI)

Isoelectric pH (pI) is the pH at which protein is in zwitter ion form (net change is neutral). Hence, if the pH of solution which contain protein is brought to isoelectric point (pI), the protein will precipitate.

Albumin which is the most common protein excreted in urine has got pI of 4.7 and urine pH is 6.5. So, adding acid in the urine drop by drop may bring the pH of urine nearer to isoelectric point (pI) of albumin (4.7) and hence albumin may get precipitated.

TEST FOR BILE PIGMENTS (FOUCHET'S TEST)

Conjugated bilirubin is soluble in plasma and gets filtered in urine. Unconjugated bilirubin is not as such soluble in plasma and tend to bind with albumin for its transportation and does not get filtered out in urine due to its large mass when combined with albumin. Presence of bilirubin in urine suggests obstructive jaundice.

Bilirubin in urine can be detected by Fouchet's test which is described in Table 4.8.

$MgSO_4$ and $BaCl_2$ interact to produce $BaSO_4$ precipitate which adsorbs bilirubin. After filtration, when precipitate is dried on filter paper and a few drops of Fouchet's reagent (prepared by adding 10 mg of 10% $FeCl_3$ to 100 ml of 25% TCA) is added; the bilirubin is oxidized to biliverdin which gives bluish green coloration (Fig. 4.3).

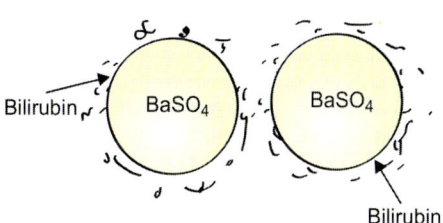

Fig. 4.3: Adsorption of bilirubin on $BaSO_4$

Table 4.8: Test for bile pigment (Fouchet's test)		
Procedure	Observation	Inference
10 mL of urine is taken in TT. 1 mL of $MgSO_4$ is added and urine is boiled. 10% $BaCl_2$ is added drop by drop to get the precipitate in tube. Filter the urine on filter paper with the help of funnel. Discard the filtrate and dry filter paper by keeping it in hot air oven at 50°C for 5 min. Add 2 drops of freshly prepared Fouchet's reagent on the ppt. Keep the filter paper in hot air oven at 50°C for 2 minutes and then observe.	Precipitate on filter paper turn bluish green	Bilirubin is present which is oxidized to biliverdin after addition of Fouchet's reagent ($FeCl_3$)

TEST FOR BILE SALT (HAY'S SULFUR TEST)

Bile salts are salts of taurocholic acid and glycocholic acid which are excreted in urine in case of obstructive jaundice.

Bile salts reduce surface tension and hence sulfur powder added in the urine sinks to bottom of test tube (Table 4.9).

TEST FOR KETONE BODY

Acetone, acetoacetic acid and beta hydroxybutyric acid are ketone bodies which are excreted in urine in condition called ketoacidosis.

Ketoacidosis may be seen as a complication of diabetes mellitus or may be a consequence of prolonged fasting and starvation.

The most common test done to detect ketone body is **Rothera's test** which detects acetone and acetoacetic acid [keto group containing ketone body]. Rothera's test does not detect β hydroxybutyrate because it lacks keto group.

For detection of β-hydroxybutyrate, modified Rothera's test is done where β hydroxybutyrate is modified to acetoacetic acid by the use of H_2O_2 and then is being tested.

Rothera's test is described in Table 4.10.

Table 4.9: Hay's sulfur test

Procedure	Observation	Inference
Two test tubes are taken; one for 'test' and another for 'control'. 'Test' TT is filled with 5 mL of urine and 'control' TT is filled with 5 mL of water. Pinch of sulfur powder is sprinkled over both the test tubes and observation made.	Sulfur powder sinks at the bottom of TT containing urine and floats on surface in TT containing water 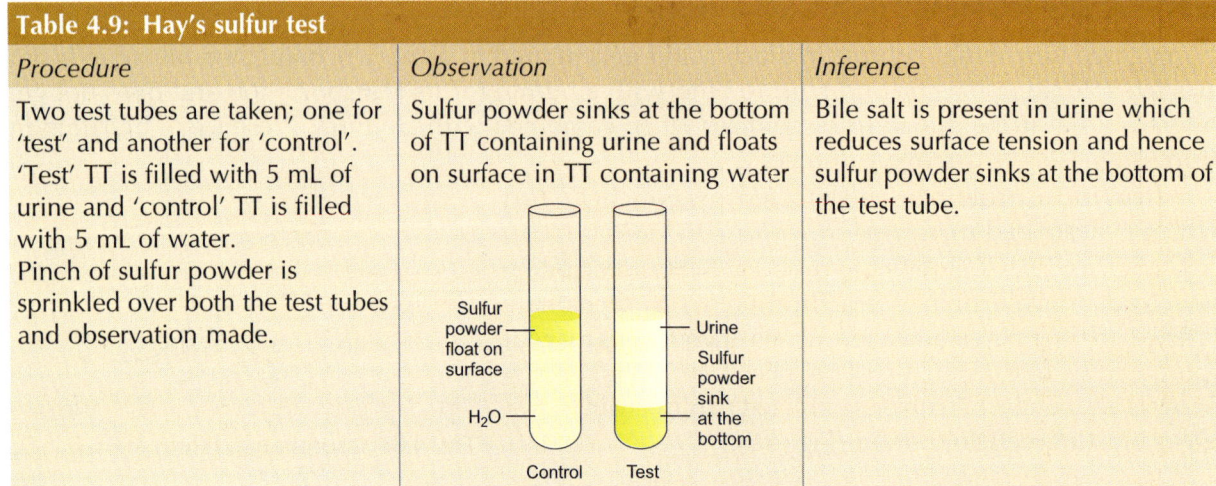	Bile salt is present in urine which reduces surface tension and hence sulfur powder sinks at the bottom of the test tube.

Note: Control tube with water is taken to check the quality of sulfur powder, if the sulfur powder floats at surface, it denotes good quality of sulfur powder and if sulfur powder sinks at the bottom of the tube containing water denotes that sulfur powder is heavy due to absorption of moisture.

Table 4.10: Rothera's test for detection of ketone bodies in the urine

Procedure	Observation	Inference
5 mL of urine is taken in TT + Saturated with ammonium sulfate* salt + 2 drops of freshly prepared 2% sodium nitroprusside is mixed in the urine +1 mL of liquor ammonia is added from the side of the tube and observation made	Purple color ring at the junction of two liquids	Presence of acetone or acetoacetic acid in the urine

*Ammonium sulfate is added to precipitate the protein in the urine.

TEST FOR DETECTION OF BLOOD (BENZIDINE TEST)

Blood in the urine is called hematuria. This is due to trauma to urinary tract or because of stone and malignancy (Table 4.11).

Table 4.11: Benzidine test to detect presence of blood in urine

Procedure	Observation	Inference
2–3 mL of urine is boiled for 5 min and then cooled. In another TT, 2–3 mL of benzidine solution is taken and equal volume of H_2O_2 is added. Boiled and cooled urine is mixed in second TT containing benzidine solution and H_2O_2, observe	Transient blue color is observed on adding the urine in test tube containing benzidine and H_2O_2	Blood is present in urine

Principle: Peroxidase activity of heme converts H_2O_2 to H_2O and nascent oxygen. Nascent oxygen acts upon benzidine to form blue-colored complex.

Benzidine is carcinogen so care should be taken for handling it.

Analysis of Abnormal Constituents in the Urine and Their Clinical Correlation

Experiment Name: Examination of urine for abnormal constituents

OBSERVATION

Physical Characteristics

Appearance: _____

Volume: _____

Color: _____

Odor: _____

pH: _____

Specific gravity: _____

Analysis of Abnormal Constituents

Experiment	Observation	Inference
Benedict's test		
Heat coagulation test		
Heller's test		
Sulfosalicylic acid test		
Fouchet's test		
Hay's sulfur test		
Rothera's test		
Benzidine test		

INTERPRETATION

Clinical Correlation: _____

_____

_____

_____

Dated: _____   **Teacher's Signature**

Experiment Name: Examination of urine for abnormal constituents

OBSERVATION

Physical Characteristics

Appearance: _____

Volume: _____

Color: _____

Odor: _____

pH: _____

Specific gravity: _____

Analysis of Abnormal Constituents

Experiment	Observation	Inference
Benedict's test		
Heat coagulation test		
Heller's test		
Sulfosalicylic acid test		
Fouchet's test		
Hay's sulfur test		
Rothera's test		
Benzidine test		

INTERPRETATION

Clinical Correlation: _____

_____

_____

_____

Dated: _____   **Teacher's Signature**

Analysis of Abnormal Constituents in the Urine and Their Clinical Correlation

Experiment Name: Examination of urine for abnormal constituents

OBSERVATION

Physical Characteristics

Appearance: _____

Volume: _____

Color: _____

Odor: _____

pH: _____

Specific gravity: _____

Analysis of Abnormal Constituents

Experiment	Observation	Inference
Benedict's test		
Heat coagulation test		
Heller's test		
Sulfosalicylic acid test		
Fouchet's test		
Hay's sulfur test		
Rothera's test		
Benzidine test		

INTERPRETATION

Clinical Correlation: _____

_____

_____

_____

Dated: _____   **Teacher's Signature**

VIVA VOCE

Q1. What is the principle of Benedict's test?

Ans. "Benedict's test" is based on reducing property of sugars. Reducing sugar reduces cupric ion (Cu^{++}) of copper sulfate to cuprous ion (Cu^+) which forms cuprous oxide (Cu_2O) which gives different shades of color based on the quantity of cuprous oxide.

Q2. Why the Benedict's test is said to be semiquantitative test?

Ans. This test is **"semiquantitative test"** because the color, which is developed, gives the appropriate value of reducing sugar in the urine.

Q3. What other compounds other than reducing sugars give Benedict test positive?

Ans. In addition to reducing sugars, certain non-carbohydrate substances also give this test positive. These substances are:
- Vitamin C (ascorbic acid)
- Homogentisic acid (HGA)
- Creatinine
- Uric acid
- Salicylates

Q4. What are the criteria of protein solubility?

Ans. There are three factors which are important for protein solubility:
  i. Intact tertiary structure of protein
  ii. Net change on the particle
  iii. Shell of hydration around it

Q5. What is principle of Heller's test?

Ans. Conc. HNO_3 is a strong denaturant. It tends to denature the protein once it comes in contact with it. Protein tends to get precipitated because of denaturation.

Q6. What is isoelectric pH?

Ans. Isoelectric pH (pI) is the pH at which protein is in zwitter ion form (net change is neutral). Hence, if the pH of solution which contains protein is brought to isoelectric point (pI), the protein will precipitate.

Q7. What is Hay's sulfur test?

Ans. Bile salts reduce surface tension and hence sulfur powder added in the urine sinks to bottom of test tube. Hence, this test is used to find out presence or absence of bile salt in the urine.

Q8. How do you test ketone body in the urine?

Ans. The most common test done to detect ketone body is Rothera's test which detects acetone and acetoacetic acid [keto group containing ketone body]. Rothera's test does not detect β hydroxybutyrate because it lacks keto group.

Notes

Notes

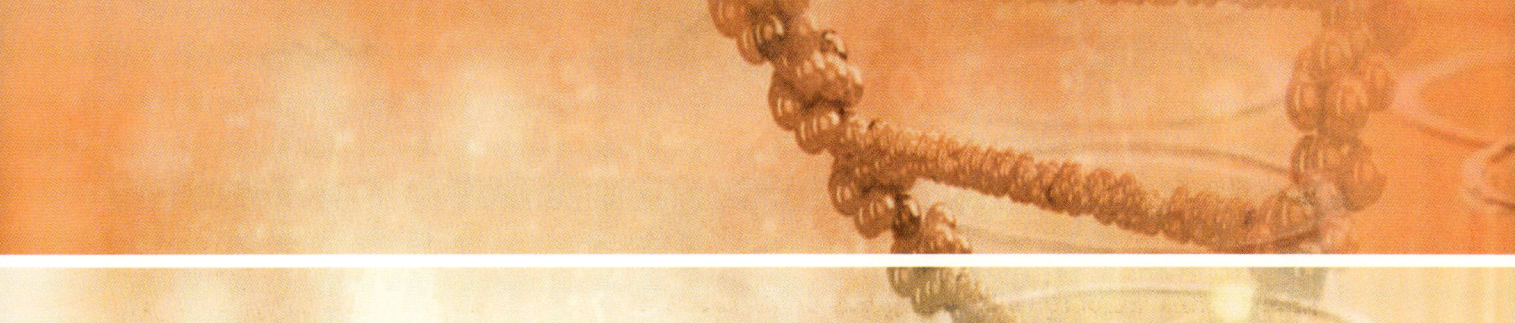

Section III

Quantitative Analysis

5. Colorimeter and Spectrophotometer: Principle and Their Functioning
6. Estimation of Glucose in Serum and Other Biological Fluids
7. Kidney Function Test: An Overview
8. Estimation of Urea in Serum and Other Biological Fluids
9. Estimation of Creatinine in Serum and Other Biological Fluids
10. Estimation of Uric Acid in Serum
11. Liver Function Test: An Overview
12. Estimation of Bilirubin
13. Estimation of AST/SGOT
14. Estimation of SGPT (ALT)
15. Estimation of ALP
16. Estimation of Total Protein in Serum and Other Biological Fluids
17. Estimation of Albumin in Serum and Calculation of A:G Ratio
18. Estimation of Total Cholesterol
19. Estimation of Triacylglycerol and HDL
20. Estimation of Calcium
21. Estimation of Phosphorus

CHAPTER

5

Colorimeter and Spectrophotometer: Principle and Their Functioning

Competencies

BI 11.6: Describe the principles of colorimetry.
BI 11.18: Discuss the principles of spectrophotometry.

COLORIMETER

It is an instrument which measures the concentration of a color complex produced via interaction of an "analyte" with a reagent or reagents (Fig. 5.1).

The amount/concentration of colored complex formed is directly proportional to the amount of targeted analyte and hence the *absorbance of light* in the colored solution is directly proportional to the concentration of targeted analyte. *Transmittance light* is inversely proportional to absorbance of light and hence to concentration of targeted analyte.

In colorimeter, the *transmittance light* is measured and is calculated for absorbance. Unit of absorbance is OD (Figs 5.2 and 5.3).

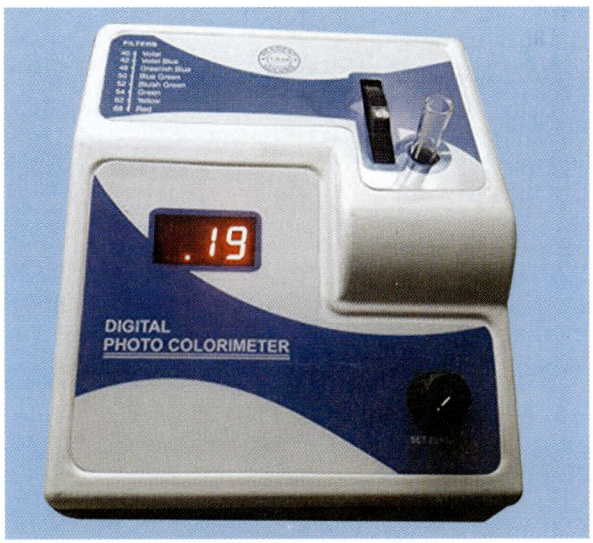

Fig. 5.1: Colorimeter

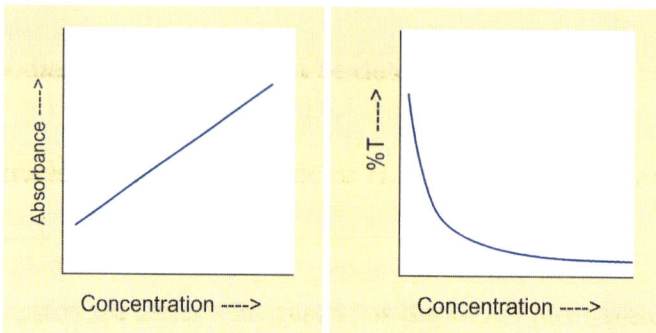

Fig. 5.2: Graphical representation of absorbance *vs* concentration and % transmittance *vs* concentration

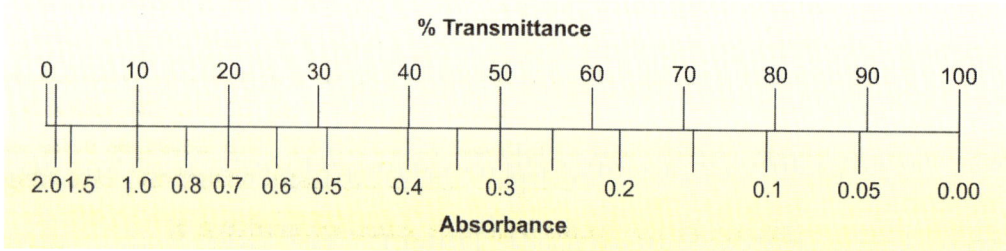

Fig. 5.3: Inverse relation of absorbance and % transmittance

Relation between absorbance and percent transmission (Fig. 5.4):
1. A = 2-log % T
   A = Absorbance
   T = Transmittance
2. A = –log T

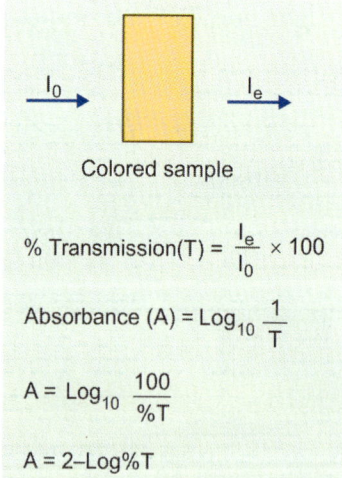

Fig. 5.4: Relation between absorbance and % transmission

COLORIMETER vs SPECTROPHOTOMETER

Both the instruments act on same principle and are used to measure the concentration of an analyte which is converted to colored complex by interaction of one or more reagents. The color

complex need not to be produced when measurement by spectrophotometer is done in ultraviolet and infrared range.
- The difference lies in the range of wavelength which can be used in these instruments. Colorimeter uses lights of visible portion of spectrum, whereas spectrophotometer uses ultraviolet, visible, infrared portion of the spectrum.

  Accordingly, tungsten bulb which emits a continuous spectrum of light in visible range (400 to 760 nm) is used in colorimeter and hydrogen or deuterium lamp which emits spectrum of light in the range of 200 to 900 nm is being used in spectrophotometer.
- *Colorimeter uses filter* to select the narrow wavelength of light, while *spectrophotometer uses prism or grating* to select monochromatic light.
- Spectrophotometer measurement is more sensitive and more accurate.

  Both these instruments are based on the principle of two laws:
  1. Lambert's law
  2. Beer law

Lambert's Law

This law states that the **optical density (absorbance)** of colored solution is directly proportional to the **path length** of the light thorough the colored solution. [Path length (b) of the light is nothing but is the diameter of the tube, i.e. the distance travelled by the light through that colored solution.]

$A \alpha b$

Beer's Law

This law states that the **optical density (absorbance)** of colored solution is directly proportional to the **(c) concentration of colored complex** which in turn is directly proportional to the concentration of analyte.

In other words, Beer's law states that concentration of substance is directly proportional to the amount of light absorbed or inversely proportional to the logarithm of the transmitted light.

$A \alpha c$

When above two laws are combined, we get following equation:

$A \alpha b \times c$

Or

$$A = abc$$

Where

        A = absorbance
        a = absorption coefficient
        b = path length in cm (tube diameter)
        c = concentration of analyte (g/dL)

[If b is 1 cm and c is expressed in moles per liter, the symbol epsilon (ϵ) is substituted for (a)]. [Epsilon (ϵ) is called molar absorptivity.]

Basic Components of Colorimeter/Spectrophotometer

Following are the basic components of a colorimeter.
1. Source of light
2. Entrance slit
3. Spectral isolation (filter/monochromator)
4. Exit slit

5. Cuvette
6. Photodetector
7. Galvanometer (readout device)

1. Source of Light
- It may be tungsten bulb which emits a continuous spectrum of light in visible range (400 to 760 nm).
- Hydrogen or deuterium lamp emits spectrum of light in the range of 200 to 900 nm (Fig. 5.5).

2. Entrance Slit
This is an arrangement for selecting narrow 'beam' of parallel light.

3. Spectral Isolation (Monochromator)
- It is done by monochromator, a device which selectively allows the monochromatic light to pass through and exclude other wavelength light.
- Monochromator may be filter (colored glass), prism or diffraction grating.
- Slits also may be inserted before and after the monochromator to achieve parallel light. Filter (colored glass) is not a true monochromator as it transmits the light over a wide range of wavelength. It is used in colorimeter.
- Prism separates white light into continuous spectrum which results in non-linear spectrum.
- A diffraction grating is prepared through deposition of aluminum-copper alloy over the flat glass plate with many lines grooves on it. Advantage of diffraction grating over the prism is that we get linear spectrum.
- Prism and grating are used in spectrophotometer.
- The wavelength of light selected for measurement of color intensity depends upon the color itself and Table 5.1 summarizes the preferred wavelength for measurement of color.

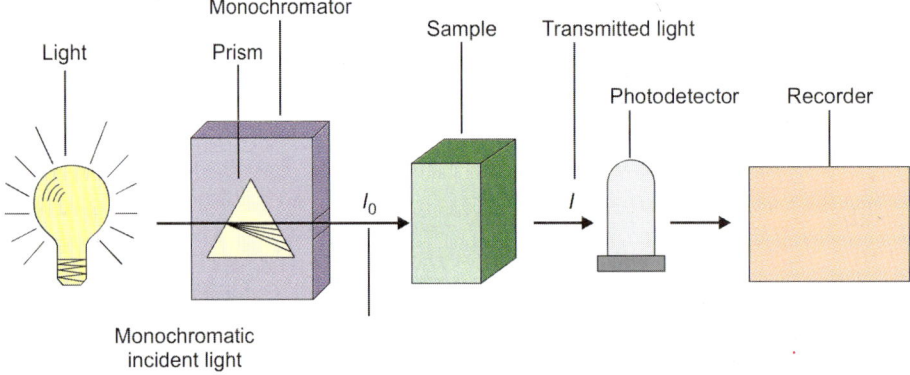

Fig. 5.5: Schematic representation of colorimeter

Table 5.1: Color scheme for colorimeter		
Color of solution	Filter to select [complimentary color]	Wavelength of light (nm)
Yellow	Blue	490
Purple	Green	530
Blue	Yellow	570
Greenish blue	Orange	600
Bluish green	Red	700 and beyond

4. Exit Slit

As mentioned previously, it helps in getting narrow and parallel beam of light.

5. Cuvette

- It is also called absorption cell and may be made up of glass, silica (quartz) or plastic. It may be round, square, or rectangular.
- For visible portion of spectrum, ordinary **borosilicate glass** is adequate; but if the reading is taken below 340 nm, **quartz cuvette** is required.
- **Plastic cuvettes** can be used for both UV and visible spectrum but they have inherent problem of temperature deformation and solvent etching. They are designed for disposable/single use application.
- Cuvette should be cleaned after use by soaking them in a mixture of **HCl: water: ethanol (1:3:4)**.

6. Photodetector

Photodetector converts light into electric energy.

7. Readout Device

The electric energy from the detector is read out either directly or after amplification. Following are certain readout devices:
- Galvanometer
- Digital readout devices
  Adjustment can be made to read the transmittance and convert it to absorbance.

VIVA VOCE

Q1. What is the relation between absorbance and transmittance of light?
Ans. Transmittance light is inversely proportional to absorbance of light.

Q2. What are the criteria of selection of filter for measurement of color in a color solution?
Ans. Complimentary color filter need to be selected which shows maximal absorption and minimal transmittance of light.

Q3. What is the equation which denotes the relation of absorbance and transmittance?
Ans. Equation is
$A = 2 - \log \% T$

Q4. What is Lambert's law?
Ans. Lambert's law states that the optical density (absorbance) of colored solution is directly proportional to the path length of the light thorough the colored solution. (Path length (b) of the light is nothing but is the diameter of the tube, i.e. the distance travelled by the light through that colored solution.)
$A \propto b$

Q5. What is Beer's law?
Ans. Beer's law states that the optical density (absorbance) of colored solution is directly proportional to the concentration of colored complex which in turn is directly proportional to the concentration of analyte.
$A \propto c$

Q6. How to measure the absorbance in invisible range?
Ans. Spectrophotometer is used to measure the absorbance in UV and infrared range?

Q7. What lamp emits lights in ultraviolet and infrared range?
Ans. Hydrogen and deuterium lamps emit lights in UV and IR range.

Q8. What is OD?
Ans. Unit of absorbance is OD.

Q9. What is the difference between colorimeter and spectrophotometer?
Ans. Colorimeter uses filter to select the narrow wavelength of light, while spectrophotometer uses prism or grating to select monochromatic light.

Notes

CHAPTER

6

Estimation of Glucose in Serum and Other Biological Fluids

Competency

BI 11.21: Demonstrate estimation of glucose in serum.

Glucose can be estimated in blood, urine and CSF.

Preferred Sample
- Plasma is preferred than serum or whole blood sample.
- Sodium fluoride and potassium oxalate is used in grey-colored capped vacutainer to collect the blood for plasma glucose estimation.
- Capillary (arterialized) blood glucose and venous blood show minor difference in fasting state; but in fed state, there is considerable variation in capillary (arterialized) blood glucose and venous blood. (Capillary blood may show 30–35 mg/dL higher glucose compared to venous blood in fed state.)
- Estimation of blood glucose is important not only to diagnose diabetes but also it gives important information regarding effectiveness of the treatment and response to therapy.
- Blood glucose estimation also helps in diagnosis of hypoglycemia which requires immediate attention.

There are broadly two important methods for estimation of glucose:
1. **Chemical methods** are the obsolete methods of glucose estimation and are based on reducing tendency of glucose. There are two methods under this heading:
   - Modified King and Asatoor method
   - Ortho-toluidine method
2. **Enzymatic method** of blood glucose estimation is more accurate and specific compared to chemical methods as the enzymes specifically act on glucose.

Either of glucose oxidase, hexokinase, glucose dehydrogenase is used, and the reaction is coupled with a reaction which produces colored substance the concentration of which is directly proportional to glucose level in the biological fluid.

All above methods are described below.

CHEMICAL METHOD

Modified King and Asatoor Method

Principle

This method is based on reducing property of glucose in alkaline medium. Glucose is heated in alkaline medium which produces enediol form, which has the tendency to reduce Cu^{++} (ic) to Cu^{+} (ous) which precipitates as insoluble cuprous oxide (Cu_2O).

Cu_2O then reduces phosphomolybdate to molybdenum blue which is measured at 610 nm. Amount of molybdenum blue is directly proportional to amount of Cu_2O, which in turn is directly proportional to amount of glucose in the solution.

Following are the reagent requirement:
- Isotonic $CuSO_4$ solution
- 10% sodium tungstate solution
- Alkaline $CuSO_4$ solution
- Phosphomolybdic acid reagent
- Glucose standard: 10 mg%

Preparation of Protein Free Filtrate (PFF) (Test Tube A)

7.4 mL of $CuSO_4$ +0.2 mL of whole blood + 0.4 mL of sodium tungstate is taken in a centrifuge tube (total 8 mL) and is mixed well. It is centrifuged at 3,000 rpm for 3 minutes, and supernatant is used for glucose estimation which is free of protein (protein free filtrate).

Procedure

Three test tubes (preferably Folin Wu tubes) are taken and marked as B (blank), S (standard) and T (test). Reagents are added as per Table 6.1.

- All the test tubes are plugged with cotton ball and are kept at boiling water bath for 10 minutes.
- After 10 minutes, tubes are removed and cooled at room temperature.
- 3 mL of phosphomolybdic acid is added followed by 8 mL of DW in each of three tubes. Solution in each test tube is thoroughly mixed by inverting the test tube over palm firmly (Fig. 6.1).
- OD reading of the solution taken at 610 nm.

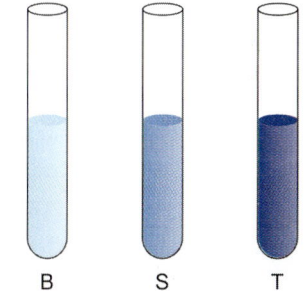

Fig. 6.1: King and Asatoor method for glucose estimation

Table 6.1: Scheme detail for glucose quantification by modified King and Asatoor method			
Reagents	B (blank) mL	S (standard) mL	T (test) mL
Distilled water (DW)	2	1.5	
Standard (10 mg %)		0.5	
PFF			2
Alkaline $CuSO_4$	2	2	2
Total	4	4	4

Calculation

Amount of glucose = OD of test/OD of standard × amount of standard/volume of serum × 100

OD of test/OD of standard × 0.05/0.05 × 100

OD of test/OD of standard × 1 × 100

[Amount of standard: 100 mL has 10 mg so 0.5 mL has 0.05 mg.]

[8 mL of solution prepared in test tube A contains 0.2 mL of blood, so 2 mL of PFF contains 0.05 mL of serum.]

Ortho-Toluidine Method

Principle

Blue green color N-glycosylamine derivative is formed when glucose interacts with ortho-toluidine in glacial acetic acid at 100°C. Intensity of this colour is directly proportional to the concentration of glucose in the solution and is read at 600 nm (red) or 630 nm (orange).

Reagents Required

1. 10% trichloroacetic acid
2. O-Toluidine reagent [5 g of thiourea is dissolved in 90 mL of O-toluidine and is made up to 1 litre with glacial acetic acid and is stored in brown bottle.)
3. Glucose standard: 10 mg%.

Procedure

Step 1: Following are taken in a test tube: 0.5 mL of blood sample, 3 mL of DW, 1.5 mL of 10% trichloroacetic acid [total 5 mL]
Mixed and kept aside for 10 min.
Filtered and used in step 2. (5 mL of this solution contains 0.5 mL of serum so 1 mL has 0.1 mL of serum.)

Step 2: Reagents are added as per scheme given in Table 6.2. Mix thoroughly and keep in boiling water bath for 10 min. Cooled and reading taken at 600/630 nm.

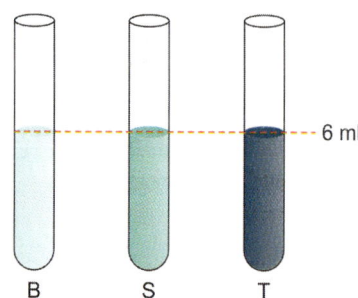

Fig. 6.2: Ortho-toluidine method for glucose estimation

Calculation

Concentration of glucose in test solution = OD of test/OD of standard × amount of standard/volume of serum × 100

OD of test/OD of standard × 0.01/0.01 × 100

OD of test/OD of standard × 1 × 100

Table 6.2: Scheme detail for glucose quantification by O-toluidine method			
Reagents	B (blank) mL	S (standard) mL	T (test) mL
DW	1		
Standard (10 mg%)		1	
Filtrate prepared in step 1			1
O-toluidine reagent	5	5	5
Total	**6**	**6**	**6**

Estimation of Glucose in Serum and Other Biological Fluids

ENZYMATIC METHOD

Glucose Oxidase Method

Principle

Aldehyde group of β-D-glucose is oxidised by glucose oxidase to produce gluconic acid. H_2O_2 is produced as byproduct in this reaction.

Rxn 1: H_2O_2 is then acted upon by peroxidase to produce nascent oxygen which interacts with dye 4-aminoantipyrine (AAP) which gives pink-colored complex of quinoneimine.

Rxn 2: Pink color is read colorimetrically at 540 nm and color absorbance (OD) is directly proportional to the amount of nascent oxygen which in turn is directly proportional to the amount of glucose in biological fluid.

$$\text{Glucose} \xrightarrow{\text{GOD}} \text{Gluconic acid} + H_2O_2$$

$$H_2O_2 \xrightarrow{\text{POD}} H_2O + [O] \text{ nascent oxygen}$$

$$\text{4-Amino antipyrine (4 AAP)} \longrightarrow \text{Quinoneimine (Pink-colored complex)}$$

Reagents Required

1. Enzyme reagent (consists of glucose oxidase, peroxidase, dye 4-aminoantipyrine (AAP), phenol in phosphate buffer.
2. Glucose standard: 100 mg%.

Procedure

Reagents are added as per plan given in Table 6.3. Mixed properly and reading is taken at 540 nm in colorimeter and OD recorded (Fig. 6.3).

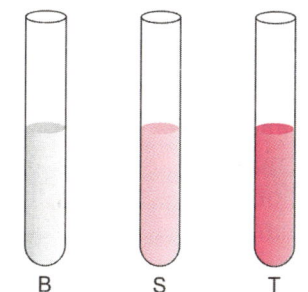

Fig. 6.3: Glucose oxidase-peroxidase [GOD-POD] method of glucose estimation

Calculation

Amount of glucose = OD of test/OD of standard × amount of standard (in mg)/volume of serum (in mL) × 100

  OD of test/OD of standard × 0.02/0.02 × 100

  OD of test/OD of standard × 1 × 100

Interference of GOD-POD method: Uric acid, glutathione, and ascorbic acid interfere with the action of glucose oxidase (GOD) enzyme.

Table 6.3: Scheme detail for glucose quantification by glucose oxidase-peroxidase(GOD-POD) method			
Reagents	B (blank)	S (standard)	T (test)
Enzyme reagent	2 mL	2 mL	2 mL
Standard (100 mg%)		20 μL	
Plasma			20 μL
DW	20 μL		

Hexokinase Method

This is the **reference method** for glucose estimation as it incorporates use of glucose-6-phosphate dehydrogenase enzyme which specifically acts on glucose-6-phosphate moiety alone.

Rxn: Glucose is acted upon by hexokinase to produce glucose-6-phosphate, which is then acted upon by glucose 6 phosphate dehydrogenase (G6PD). G6PD converts G6P to 6-phosphogluconate with concomitant release of NADPH.

NADPH produced is directly proportional to the amount of glucose. NADPH absorbs wavelength at 340 nm and can be quantified by increase in absorbance at 340 nm.

Clinistix Test

In this, an area on the stick is impregnated with o-toluidine, glucose oxidase, and a pink background dye. It is dipped in test-tube containing 5 mL urine for 10 seconds and if stick area turns shades of blue, it denotes presence of glucose in urine (glucose concentration should be above 1 g/L).

O-toluidine is oxidized to a blue substance which gives various shades of blue.

> **Competency**
>
> **IM11.12:** Perform and interpret a capillary blood glucose test.

Self-monitoring of blood glucose (SMBG) is an important concept which helps patients to monitor their blood glucose level and modulate the dose of insulin accordingly under the supervision of clinician.

Portable machine known as glucometer is a popular instrument in this regard which gives accurate information regarding capillary blood glucose level. This instrument is commonly being used not only by physician at his clinic and hospitals as a bedside measure of blood glucose monitoring, it is also a common household item which is extensively used by patient himself to estimate blood glucose (Fig. 6.4).

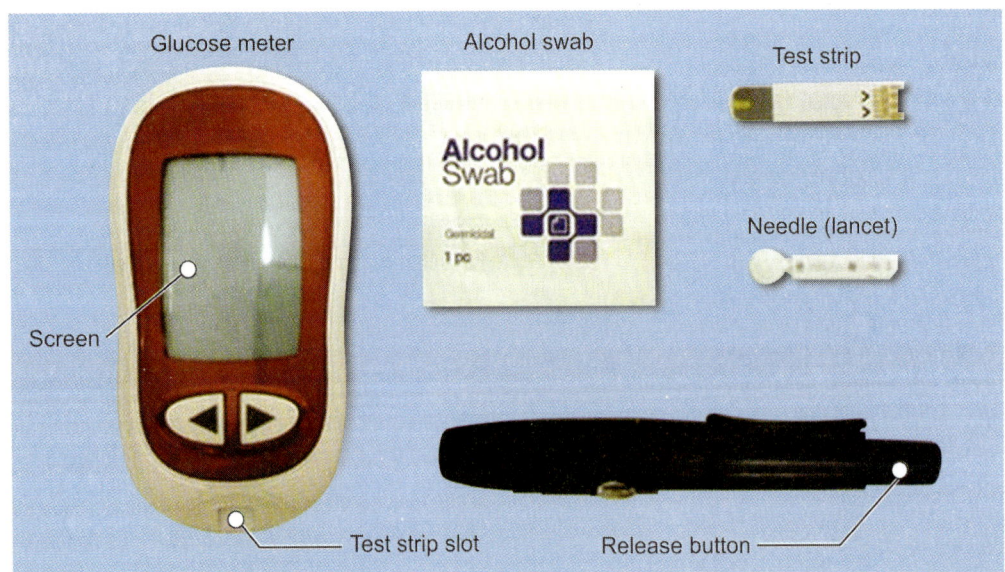

Fig. 6.4: Glucometer instrument and its accessories

This instrument is based on the principles of enzymatic assessment of blood glucose. The kit of glucometer contains following items in it:
- Instrument glucometer
- Test strips
- Needle (Lancet)
- Lancet device
- Alcohol swab

Strips of glucometer are specially designed to contain enzyme in dry form at one of its ends (glucose oxidase-peroxidase). A drop of capillary arterial blood from fingerprick is placed carefully at designated spot and it is allowed to react with the enzyme in the strip.

Strip is then inserted in the glucometer in a direction specific manner. In some of the glucometer instrument, strip is first inserted into the glucometer instrument and then the blood sample is applied as a second step as shown in the Fig. 6.5.

After a fixed period of time which may vary from 5 to 45 seconds, reading appears in digital display screen.

Variability in terms of sample required (may vary from 0.3 to 1.5 microliter), test time incubation (may range from 5 to 45 sec) and the range of values which can be measured (0 to 600 mg/dL to 30 to 500 mg/dL) is noticed in various glucometers of different manufacturers.

It is important to note that the sample used in this instrument is whole blood. Whole blood glucose concentration is 10 to 15% lower than the plasma or serum glucose concentration.

Manufacturers may calibrate the instrument to give the result of plasma glucose, even if the sample used is whole blood.

Steps to Perform Glucose Estimation using Glucometer (Fig. 6.5)

1. Switch on the machine.
2. Place the test strip in the socket correctly.
3. Clean the fingertip with alcohol swab (any fingertip may be selected).

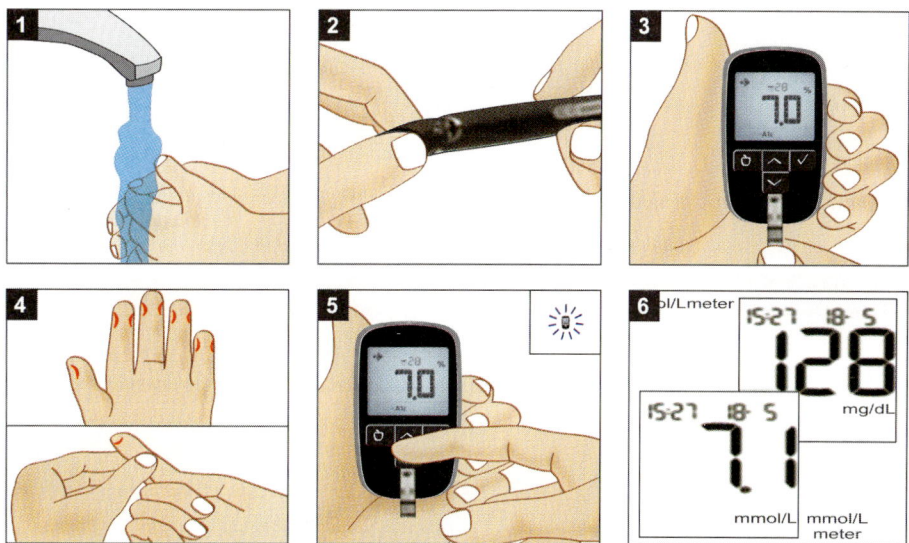

Fig. 6.5: Steps to perform glucose estimation using glucometer

4. Place the lancet in lancet holder.
5. Prick the finger with desired force which can be adjusted in the lancet holder.
6. Put a drop of blood at correct spot and wait for the result.
7. Read the result at the screen and remove and dispose the test strip.

Diastix

In this, an area on the stick is impregnated with potassium iodide, glucose oxidase, and a blue background dye. It is dipped in test-tube containing 5 mL urine for 30 seconds and if stick area changes colour in varying shades of green to blue, it denotes presence of glucose in urine.

Glycosylated Hemoglobin (HbA1c)

- Non-enzymatic glycosylation of beta chain N-terminal valine amino acid with glucose results in formation of HbA1c.
- Quantity of HbA1c is represented as percentage of total hemoglobin, hence its unit is % (not gram%).
- As the life of RBC is 120 days, measurement of HbA1c gives idea about average blood sugar in preceding 8–12 weeks.
- HbA1a, HbA1b and HbA1c collectively known as glycated hemoglobin (Tables 6.4 and 6.5).
- Cation exchange chromatography is routinely used for measurement of HbA1c.
- Single value of 6.5% in random blood sample is sufficient for the diagnosis of diabetes mellitus as per latest consensus.
- HbA1c measurement is also useful to know the patient compliance to the treatment as well as the effectiveness of therapy being implemented in diabetic patient.

Table 6.4: Various types of glycated hemoglobin	
Type of glycated hemoglobin	Compound which binds
HbA1a1	Fructose 1, 6-bisphosphate
HbA1a2	Glucose-6-phosphate
HbA1b	Pyruvic acid
*HbA1c	Glucose

*HbA1c is useful to know the status of diabetic patient.

Table 6.5: HbA1c and diabetic status	
HbA1c	Status
<5.7%	Non-diabetic
5.7–6.4%	Prediabetic
≥6.5%	Diabetes
<7%	Goal of therapy
>8%	Action suggested

HbA1c can be calculated for mean plasma glucose as per following protocol given in Table 6.6 [*rule of 8]

Table 6.6: HbA1c and corresponding mean plasma [*Rule of 8]	
HbA1c	Mean plasma glucose (mg%)
5	75
6	110
7	145
8	**180 mg%**
9	215

*Rule of 8: According to this, for HbA1c value of 8%, mean plasma value is taken as 180 mg% and for every 1% increase or decrease of HbA1c, 35 mg% of glucose is added or subtracted respectively from 180 mg% value to get the mean plasma glucose value.

Estimation of Glucose

Method Used: _____
_____
_____
_____

Observation

OD of test: _____

OD of standard: _____

Calculation

Concentration of glucose in serum (mg/dL) =

OD of test/OD of standard × amount of standard/volume of serum × 100

Result

_____
_____
_____

Clinical Correlation: _____
_____
_____
_____

Dated: _____   **Teacher's Signature**

Estimation of Glucose in Serum and Other Biological Fluids

Estimation of Glucose

Method Used: _____
_____
_____
_____

Observation

OD of test: _____

OD of standard: _____

Calculation

Concentration of glucose in serum (mg/dL) =

OD of test/OD of standard × amount of standard/volume of serum × 100

Result

_____
_____
_____

Clinical Correlation: _____
_____
_____
_____

Dated: _____   **Teacher's Signature**

VIVA VOCE

Q1. What are all methods you know to quantitatively estimate glucose in any biological fluid?

Ans. Following methods can be used:
- Glucose oxidase-peroxidase method
- King and Asatoor method
- Hexokinase method
- Ortho-toluidine method

Q2. What is the best method you know for glucose estimation and why?

Ans. Enzymatic methods are best because they specifically act at glucose.

Q3. Which sample (whole blood/plasma or serum) is preferred for glucose estimation and why?

Ans. Plasma is preferred then serum or whole blood sample.

Q4. What are antiglycolytic and anticoagulant most commonly being used to collect the blood for glucose estimation?

Ans. Sodium fluoride as antiglycolytic agent and potassium oxalate as anticoagulant are used.

Q5. What is the color of cap of vacutainer used for blood collection for glucose measurement?

Ans. Gray color cap

Q6. Name the pink-colored complex formed in GOD-POD method.

Ans. Quinoneimine complex

Q7. What is the wavelength light used in measuring the pink color developed in GOD-POD method and why?

Ans. Pink-colored complex reading is taken at 540 nm in colorimeter because 540 nm is complimentary wavelength for pink color and it shows maximum absorbance.

Q8. How do you define hypoglycemia?

Ans. Blood glucose level of <40 mg/dL is defined as hypoglycemia.

Q9. In a healthy person, what metabolic pathway provides glucose in the blood during hypoglycemia?

Ans.
- Glycogenolysis (liver)
- Gluconeogenesis

Q10. What are all the ways by which insulin lower the blood glucose level?

Ans. Insulin lower the blood glucose level by following means.
a. Enhancing uptake of glucose by cells
b. Enhancing glycolysis in liver
c. Enhancing glycogenesis in liver

Q11. What are the ADA criteria for diagnosis of diabetes?
Ans.

American Diabetes Association (ADA) diagnostic criteria for diabetes		
Test	Threshold	Qualifier
Hemoglobin A1c or	≥6.5%	Lab NGSP-certified, standardized DCCT assay
Fasting glucose or	≥126 mg/dL (7.0 mmol/L)	No caloric intake for at least 8 hours
2-hour glucose or	≥200 mg/dL (11.1 mmol/L)	After 75 g of anhydrous glucose
Random glucose	≥200 mg/dL (11.1 mmol/L)	Plus classic hyperglycemia symptoms or crisis

NGSP, National Glycohemoglobin Standardization Program; DCCT, Diabetes Control and Complications Trial.
*Results must be confirmed by repeated testing.

Q12. What do you mean by fasting blood sample?
Ans. Blood collected after 8 to 12 hrs of fasting gives fasting glucose value.

Q13. What is impaired fasting glucose?
Ans. If the fasting blood glucose is >100 mg/dL but <126 mg/dL, it is called impaired fasting glucose.

Q14. What is impaired glucose tolerance?
Ans. If the blood glucose 2 hr after intake of glucose is >140 mg/dL and <200 mg/dL, it is called impaired glucose tolerance.

Q15. What is the unit of HbA1c measurement?
Ans. It is represented as % of total hemoglobin.

Q16. What is the difference between glycated hemoglobin and glycosylated hemoglobin?
Ans. Non-enzymatic glycosylation of beta chain N-terminal valine amino acid with glucose results in formation of glycosylated hemoglobin (HbA1c).
HbA1a, HbA1b and HbA1c collectively known as glycated hemoglobin.

Q17. Estimation of HbA1c gives record of mean blood glucose of how many months duration?
Ans. As the life of RBC is 120 days, measurement of HbA1c gives idea about average blood sugar in preceding 8–12 weeks.

Q18. Which sample (arterial/venous/capillary) is preferred for routine biochemistry analysis?
Ans. Venous sample collected from antecubital vein is most commonly used sample for routine biochemistry measurement.

Q19. What is hypoglycemia? Mention few causes of hypoglycemia.
Ans. Hypoglycemia is when plasma glucose level is below 40 mg/dL. Conditions where hypoglycemia is seen are
- Various types of glycogen storage disorder which adversely affect glycogenolysis in the liver
- Overdose of insulin
- Starvation
- Insulinoma which is tumor of beta cell pancreas.

Notes

CHAPTER 7

Kidney Function Test: An Overview

> **Competencies**
>
> **BI 6.14 [A to D]:** Describe the tests that are commonly done in clinical practice to assess the functions of kidney.
> **PY 7.8:** Describe and discuss renal function tests.

Tests which are being done to assess the various aspect of kidney functioning are collectively known as kidney function test.

Broadly, kidney function tests are classified into:
- Glomerular function test
- Tubular function test

Glomerular function test includes the tests which assess:
- Functioning of glomerulus in terms of **filtration capacity** like the estimation of blood urea, serum creatinine, serum uric acid and various clearance tests, and
- The tests designed to **assess the intactness of basement membrane**, e.g. tests for proteinuria, hematuria, etc.

Tubular function test includes the tests which assess:
- Concentration test
- Dilution test

GLOMERULAR FUNCTION TEST

Test for Assessment of Glomerular Filtration Capacity

To assess the glomerular filtration capacity, following parameters are assessed in blood:
a. Blood urea
b. Serum creatinine
c. Serum uric acid
d. Clearance study

All above tests will now be described one by one. Their detailed method of assessment and clinical importance are given in Chapters 8, 9 and 10.

Blood Urea Assessment

Urea is the major nitrogenous waste substance produced during protein catabolism. It constitutes 75% of non-protein nitrogen which is excreted. Major route of urea excretion is kidney which removes 90% of total urea from the body, remaining 10% of total urea is excreted from gastrointestinal tract (GIT) and skin.

Urea is freely filtered through glomeruli, hence any dysfunction of glomeruli whereby filtration is affected, urea tends to accumulate in plasma and estimation of plasma urea gives fair idea regarding renal function.

Following methods are used for estimation of plasma urea:
1. DAM-TSC method (diacetyl monoxime-thiosemicarbazide)
2. Berthelot method.

1. **DAM-TSC method (Fearon method):** It is chemical method whereby urea is made to react with diacetyl monoaxime (DAM) in presence of ferric ion, to give pink-colored complex which is read at 540 nm (green filter) by colorimeter.

Thioemicarbazide (TSC) acts as stabilizer of color in this method.

2. **Enzymatic method [Berthelot reaction]:** It is most commonly used method for urea estimation in clinical laboratories. Urease hydrolyzes urea into ammonium ion (NH_4^+) and carbonate (CO_3^{2-}). NH_4^+ then interacts with 2-oxoglutarate in presence of glutamate dehydrogenase [GLDH] and rate of disappearance of NADH is measured at 340 nm (Fig. 7.1).

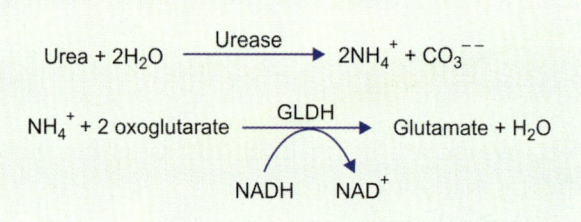

Fig. 7.1: Principle of Berthelot reaction

The released NH_4^+ can also be quantified by various other methods like:
- Color change associated with pH indicator.
- Glutamine synthetase
- Pyruvate kinase
- Pyruvate oxidase

Assessment of Serum Creatinine (Jaffe Reaction)

Proposed by Jaffe in 1886, this method is based on reaction of creatinine with picric acid in alkaline condition to give red-orange chromogen (alkaline picrate) which is read at 490 nm.

This reaction is non-specific and has positive interference by acetone, acetoacetate, glucose, ascorbate and pyruvate.

To increase the specificity of this reaction, two approaches are used:
1. Kinetic Jaffe method
2. Coupled enzymatic method (using creatininase, peroxidase, etc.) (Fig. 7.2)

Uric Acid Assessment

Following methods may be adopted to estimate uric acid in biological fluid.
- Phosphotungstic acid (PTA) [Caraway method]
- Uricase method

Phosphotungstic acid [Caraway method]: Uric acid reacts with phosphotungstic acid in alkaline medium and produces tungsten blue the absorbance of which is measured at 650 nm.

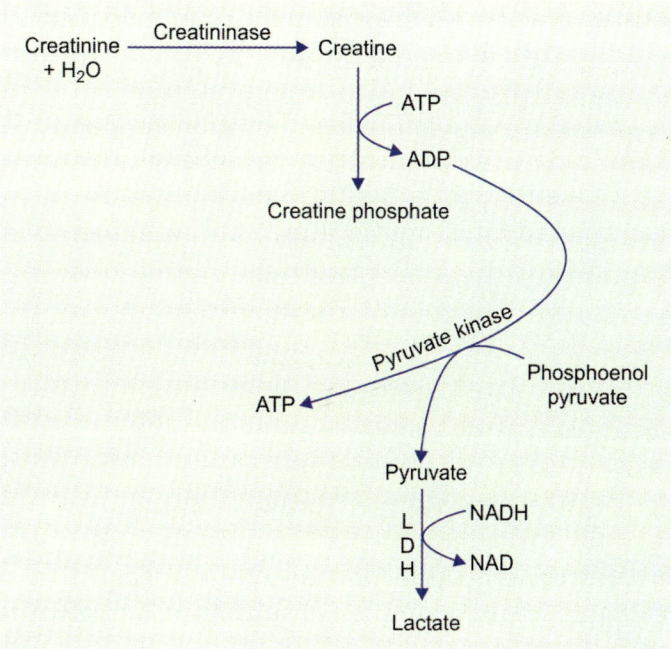

Fig. 7.2: Coupled enzymatic method for creatinine estimation

The absorbance at 650 nm is directly proportional to amount of uric acid present in biological fluid.

Uricase method [enzymatic method]: Enzyme uricase acts on uric acid to convert it to allantoin and H_2O_2. Released H_2O_2 is acted upon by peroxidase enzyme and nascent oxygen [O] is released. This nascent oxygen reacts with chromogen to produce pink-colored complex (Fig. 7.3).

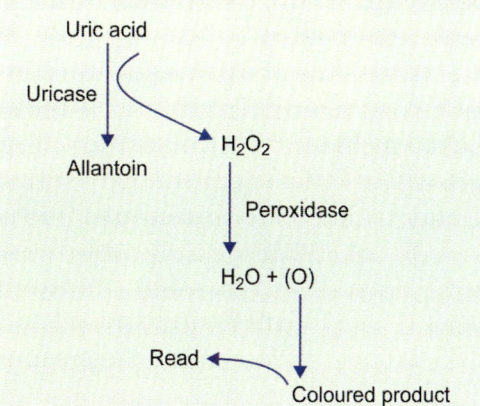

Fig. 7.3: Principle of uricase method for uric acid estimation

Clearance Study

Clearance is defined as, **"volume of plasma which is completely cleaned of a substance"** by both the kidneys in unit time.

Ideal substance for clearance study is the one which is freely filtered from glomerulus and is neither secreted nor reabsorbed from tubular epithelium. This kind of substance gives clearance, which is equal to GFR.

Inulin (exogenous substance) and to lesser extent creatinine (endogenous substance) fulfill above criteria. 40–60% of total urea which is filtered is reabsorbed, hence its clearance is lesser than the GFR.

Para-amino hippuric acid (PAH) is totally filtered by glomeruli and additionally it is secreted by tubules also, hence its clearance assessment shows higher clearance value compared to GFR. PAH clearance rather gives information regarding renal blood flow.

Substances which may be used for clearance study may be endogenous or exogenous:
A. Endogenous substances are:
- Creatinine
- Urea

B. Exogenous substances are:
- Inulin
- Iohexol
- ^{51}Cr EDTA
- ^{99m}Tc-diethylenetriamine penta-acetic acid (DTPA)

Creatinine clearance: Creatinine is endogenous excretory substance which is produced at constant rate from creatine in an individual. This substance is freely filtered at glomeruli and only minimally reabsorbed in proximal tubules; hence its clearance gives almost exact value to GFR.

$$\text{Creatinine clearance is calculated using following formula} = UV/P \text{ mL/min}$$

Where
U = urinary concentration of creatinine in mg/dL;
V = volume of urine excreted (mL) per minute;
P = plasma concentration of creatinine in mg/dL

Calculation: 24-hour urine is collected and urine excreted in each min is calculated using following formula.

Urine volume per min = Total volume of urine in 24-hour (in mL)/24 × 60

As the total content of creatine and hence the level of creatinine varies with body mass, the correction factor should ideally be included in calculation of creatinine clearance. 1.73/A is the correction factor for body mass, where A is the patient body surface area.

Hence, creatinine clearance after taking body surface area into consideration becomes

$$UV/P \times 1.73/A$$

Normal creatinine clearance: It is 100–125 mL/min in male and 90–115 mL/min in female.

After taking correction for BSA (body surface area), the creatinine clearance in both genders becomes 100 mL/min.

Creatinine clearance study helps estimating GFR and hence gives important information regarding glomerular filtration capacity.

Urea clearance study: Urea is not preferred substance for clearance study due to following reasons:
1. 40–60% of total filtered urea is reabsorbed by PCT, hence urea clearance underestimates the GFR. [Urea clearance is less than GFR.]
2. Content of urea in blood and hence its excretion (clearance) by the kidney varies with protein diet, so dietary pattern influences urea clearance study and does not accurately assess glomerular function.

Maximum urea clearance: When rate of urinary output is ≥2 mL/min, maximum urea clearance is studied by following formula:

$$UV/P \text{ [Normal is 75 mL/min]}$$

Standard urea clearance: But if the rate of urine output is <2 mL/min, standard urea clearance is studied by following formula:

$$\frac{U\sqrt{V}}{P} \text{ [Normal is 54 mL/min]}$$

Inulin clearance: Inulin is fructosan which is not metabolized by body and is freely filtered by glomeruli. It is neither secreted nor reabsorbed by kidney tubules, hence its clearance gives accurate estimate of GFR.

Inulin is an exogenous substance and should be given intravenously (IV) for GFR estimation. In addition to clearance studies described above, glomerular function is also assessed by estimation of urea and creatinine in the blood.

Assessment of Intactness of Glomerular Basement Membrane

To assess the intactness of basement membrane, following test to be done.

Proteinuria: Normal protein excretion in 24-hour urine collection is <150 mg/day; out of which albumin is <30 mg/day. If the excretion of total protein or albumin is exceeding this limit, it denotes glomerular basement membrane damage. If the total amount of albumin excreted in 24-hour urine collection is in the range of 30 to 300 mg, it denotes microalbuminuria.

Hematuria: In damage of basement membrane, RBC passes basement membrane and gets excreted in urine. It appears as RBC cast on urine microscopic examination.

TUBULAR FUNCTION TEST/ASSESSMENT (Fig. 7.4)

One of the earliest findings in tubular dysfunction is inability of tubules to concentrate the urine and passage of dilute urine.

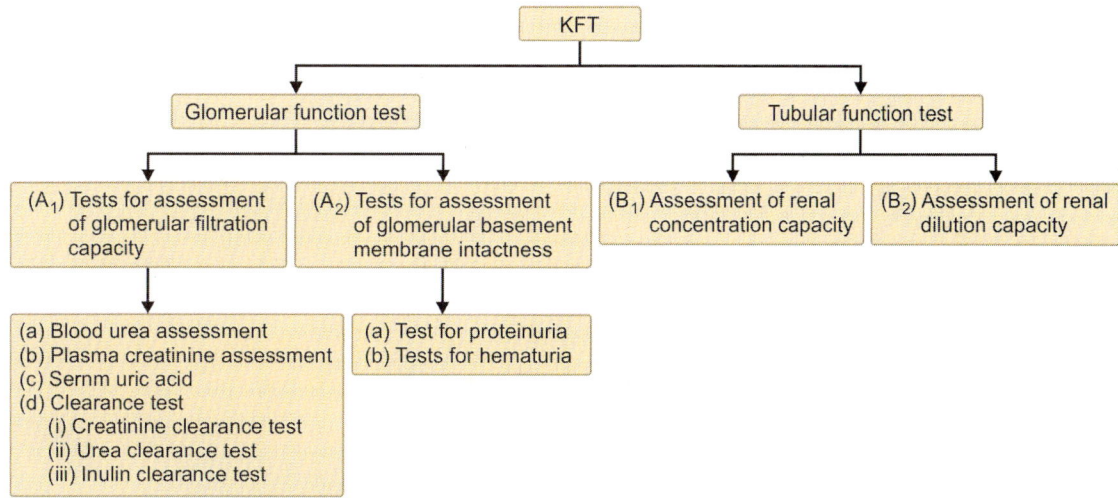

Fig. 7.4: Kidney function test: An overview

Assessment of Renal Concentration Capacity

Urinary concentration can be quantified by measuring specific gravity or by measuring urinary osmolality. Specific gravity testing is more commonly used than urinary osmolality testing, but urinary osmolality testing is more accurate than urinary specific gravity testing.

Normal urinary specific gravity is 1.010 and it can be measured by urinometer.

Urinary osmolality varies widely, depending upon the state of hydration and may range from 50 to 1400 mOsm/kg.

If after 12 hours of fluid restriction, urinary osmolality is greater than 600 mOsm/kg, it is assumed that renal concentration ability is normal.

Assessment of Renal Dilution Capacity

After overnight fast, patient is given 1000 mL of water to drink over a period of 30 minutes, after this, every hour urine sample is collected for next four hours.

Specific gravity of 1.003 or below in any one of above urinary sample denotes that tubules are functioning well.

VIVA VOCE

Q1. What are all tests included in glomerular function test?
Ans. Glomerular function test includes the tests which assess
  i. Functioning of glomerulus in terms of filtration capacity
  ii. The tests designed to assess the intactness of basement membrane

Q2. How will you assess functioning of glomerulus in terms of filtration capacity?
Ans. To assess the glomerular filtration capacity, following parameters are assessed in blood:
a. Blood urea
b. Serum creatinine
c. Serum uric acid
d. Clearance study

Q3. How will you assess the intactness of basement membrane?
Ans. To assess the intactness of basement membrane, following tests are being done:
- Test for proteinuria
- Test for hematuria

Q4. How to define clearance?
Ans. Clearance is defined as, "Volume of plasma which is completely cleaned of a substance by both the kidney in unit time".

Q5. What is an ideal substance for clearance study?
Ans. Ideal substance for clearance study is the one which is freely filtered from glomerulus and is neither secreted nor reabsorbed from tubular epithelium. This kind of substance gives clearance, which is equal to GFR.

Q6. How many types of substances can be used for clearance study?
Ans. Substances which may be used for clearance study may be endogenous or exogenous.
A. *Endogenous substances are*
- Creatinine
- Urea

B. *Exogenous substances are*
- Inulin
- Iohexol
- ^{51}Cr EDTA
- ^{99m}Tc-diethylenetriamine penta-acetic acid (DTPA)

Q7. What is the best substance among all mentioned above for studying the clearance?
Ans. Inulin is the best of all.

Q8. What is the best endogenous substance for studying the clearance?
Ans. Creatinine is the best endogenous substance for clearance study.

Q9. What is the normal amount of protein excretion in urine?
Ans. Normal protein excretion in 24-hour urine collection is <150 mg/day; out of which albumia is <30 mg/day. If the excretion of total protein or albumin is exceeding this limit, it denotes glomerular basement membrane damage.

Q10. How do you define microalbuminuria?
Ans. Normal protein excretion in 24-hour urine collection is <150 mg/day; out of which albumin is <30 mg/day 24-hour urine excretion in the range of 30–300 mg denotes microalbuminuria.

Notes

CHAPTER

8

Estimation of Urea in Serum and Other Biological Fluids

> **Competency**
>
> **BI 11.21:** Demonstrate estimation of urea in serum.

As stated in previous chapter (Chapter 7: KFT: An Overview), blood urea assessment is done to assess glomerular function test.

Urea is the end product of amino acid metabolism. Ammonia is very toxic and is converted to less toxic urea in a series of reaction in the liver which is called urea cycle. Urea is the major non-protein nitrogenous waste substance constituting >75% of it. Other non-protein nitrogenous (NPN) substances are creatinine, uric acid and ammonia.

Major route of urea excretion is kidney which removes 90% of total urea. Remaining 10% is excreted through GIT and skin.

Urea is freely filtered through glomerulus, hence any dysfunction of glomeruli whereby filtration is affected, urea tends to accumulate in plasma and estimation of plasma urea gives fair idea regarding renal function.

Following methods may be used for estimation of plasma urea:
1. DAM-TSC (diacetyl-monoxime-thiosemicarbazide) method (Fearon method)
2. Enzymatic method (Berthelot reaction)

DAM-TSC METHOD

Principle

- It is a chemical method where urea is made to react with **diacetyl-monoxime (DAM)** in presence of strong acid medium and ferric ion.
- In presence of acidic medium, diacetyl-monoxime is broken to release diacetyl and hydroxylamine.
- Diacetyl and urea interact to give pink-colored condensation product **"Diazine"** which is being read in colorimeter at 540 nm at green filter.
- **Thiosemicarbazide (TSC)** acts to intensify the color in this reaction. Initial color of the diazine is yellow, which is intensified to pink in presence of thiosemicarbazide.
- Ferric ion helps in stabilizing the color.

Reagents Required

1. Acid reagent ($FeCl_3$ in orthophosphoric acid)

2. Coloring reagent {diacetyl-monoxime (DAM) and thiosemicarbazide (TSC) in sulfuric acid}
3. Urea standard (1 mg%)

Procedure

- Three test tubes are taken and marked as B, S, T.
- Reagents are added as given in Table 8.1.
- Test tubes are shaken to mix the solution and they are placed in boiling water bath for 20 minutes. Thereafter they are cooled and OD reading is taken at 520 nm (Fig. 8.1).

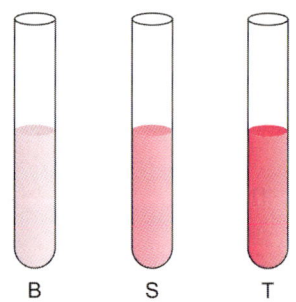

Fig. 8.1: DAM-TSC method of urea estimation

Table 8.1: Scheme detail for urea quantification by DAM-TSC method			
Reagents	B (blank) mL	S (standard) mL	T (test) mL
Standard urea [1 mg/dL]		1	
Serum [1:100 dil]			1
DW	2	1	1
Coloring reagent	2	2	2
Acid reagent	2	2	2
Total	6	6	6

Calculation

Concentration of urea in serum = OD of test/OD of standard × amount of standard (in mg)/volume of serum (in mL) × 100

OD of test/OD of standard × 0.02/0.02 × 100

OD of test/OD of standard × 1 × 100

Interpretation

Normal range of urea in a healthy adult: 15–40 mg/dL.

High urea (uremia): Seen in condition like renal failure.

Low urea:
- Seen in very low protein intake
- Extreme stage of liver disease
- Hemodilution

Serum Urea vs BUN (Blood Urea Nitrogen)

At times the level of urea is represented in BUN.

60 g of urea contains 28 g of nitrogen and hence, the **conversion factor for changing the value of urea to BUN is 0.46,** and in case **BUN is to be converted to blood urea, the conversion factor is 2.14.**

mg/dL vs mmol/L of urea concentration: Conversion factor for converting mg/dL to mmol/L is 0.357, i.e. 40 mg/dL is 40 × 0.357 = 14.28 mmol/L.

Urinary urea estimation: As there is large amount of urea is excreted in urine (30 g/day/2000 mg/dL), urine needs to be diluted 50 or 100 times before the urinary urea is estimated.

ENZYMATIC METHOD OF UREA ASSESSMENT (BERTHELOT REACTION)

It is the most commonly used method in clinical laboratories.

Principle

- In this method, the enzyme urease first hydrolyses urea into ammonium ion (NH_4) and carbonate (CO_3).
- Ammonium ion then interacts with 2-oxoglutarate in presence of glutamate dehydrogenase (GLDH) and rate of disappearance of NADH is measured at 340 nm.

Rxn

The released ammonia can also be quantified by other methods, like:
1. Color change associated with pH indicator
2. Glutamine synthetase
3. Pyruvate kinase
4. Pyruvate oxidase

For urea clearance study, reader is directed to Chapter 7 (KFT: An Overview).

Estimation of Urea

Method Used: _____
_____
_____
_____

Observation

OD of test: _____

OD of standard: _____

Calculation

Concentration of urea in serum (mg/dL) =

OD of test/OD of standard × amount of standard/volume of serum × 100

Result

_____
_____
_____

Clinical Correlation: _____
_____
_____
_____

Dated: _____   **Teacher's Signature**

Clearance Study: _____
_____

U (Urinary urea in mg/dL): _____
_____

V (Volume of urine per minute): _____
_____

P (Plasma urea in mg/dL): _____
_____

Formula

$$\text{Maximum urea clearance} = \frac{U \times V}{P}$$

$$\text{Standard urea clearance} = \frac{U \times \sqrt{V}}{P}$$

VIVA VOCE

Q1. What are the non-proteinic nitrogen substances?
Ans. They are:
- Urea
- Creatinine
- Uric acid

Q2. What is the source of urea?
Ans. Urea is the end product of amino acid metabolism.

Q3. What are NPN (non-protein nitrogenous) substances? Give examples.
Ans. NPN substances are urea, creatinine, uric acid and ammonia.

Q4. What are all methods you know which can be used for estimation of urea in biological fluid?
Ans. Following methods may be used for estimation of plasma urea:
- DAM-TSC (diacetyl-monoxime-thiosemicarbazide) method (Fearon method)
- Enzymatic method (Berthelot reaction)

Q5. What is the principle of DAM-TSC (diacetyl-monoxime-thiosemicarbazide) method?
Ans. It is a chemical method where urea is made to react with diacetyl-monoxime (DAM) in presence of strong acid medium and ferric ion. In presence of acidic medium, diacetyl-monoxime is broken to release diacetyl and hydroxylamine. Diacetyl and urea interact to give pink-colored condensation product "Diazine" which is being read in colorimeter at 540 nm at green filter.

Q6. What is the role of thiosemicarbazide (TSC) and ferric ion in DAM-TSC (diacetyl-monoxime-thiosemicarbazide) method for urea estimation?
Ans. Thiosemicarbazide (TSC) acts to intensify the color in this reaction. Initial color of the diazine is yellow, which is intensified to pink in presence of thiosemicarbazide.

Ferric ion helps in stabilizing the color.

Q7. What is the normal range of urea in a healthy adult?
Ans. Normal range of urea in a healthy adult: 15–40 mg/dL

Q8. How to interconvert the value of blood urea and BUN (blood urea nitrogen)?
Ans. Serum urea vs BUN (blood urea nitrogen):
- 60 g of urea contains 28 g of nitrogen.
- Hence, the conversion factor for changing the value of urea to BUN is 0.46.
- If BUN is to be converted to blood urea, the conversion factor is 2.14.

Q9. What is the difference between terminologies "uremia" and "azotemia"?
Ans. Azotemia is a biochemical abnormality, defined as elevation of, nitrogenous products like urea, creatinine in the blood, and other secondary waste products within the body. Raising the level of nitrogenous waste is attributed to the inability of the renal system to filter such as waste products adequately.

Azotemia when associated with clinical sign and symptoms of chronic renal failure is known as uremia. In uremia, patient has nausea, vomiting, anorexia, metallic taste in mouth along with muscular pain, characteristic odour of breath, mental confusion and acid-base disorder.

Q10. Mention causes of raised urea in blood.

Ans. Causes of azotemia may be prerenal, renal or postrenal.

Prerenal azotemia: It is due to reduced GFR which may be due to following conditions:
- Dehydration
- Shock (cardiac failure)
- Massive hemorrhage
- Burn

Renal azotemia: Renal azotemia results from decreased GFR when more than ¾ of the nephrons (glomeruli) are non-functional. Renal azotemia may be due to: Primary intrinsic renal disease (glomerulonephritis, ethylene glycol toxicity) or may be due to renal injury that occurs secondary to renal ischemia, such as from prerenal causes, or urinary tract obstruction (post-renal azotemia).

Post-renal azotemia: Post-renal azotemia results from obstruction (urolithiasis) or rupture (uroabdomen) of urinary outflow tracts.

Notes

CHAPTER

9

Estimation of Creatinine in Serum and Other Biological Fluids

> **Competencies**
>
> **BI 11.21:** Demonstrate estimation of creatinine in serum.
> **BI 11.7:** Demonstrate the estimation of serum creatinine and creatinine clearance.

Serum creatinine assessment is done to assess glomerular function test.

Creatine is the compound which is stored in the muscle in the form of creatine phosphate (phosphagen). Creatine phosphate is the instant source of ATP and provides ATP during muscle exercise. Figure 9.1 explains the role of creatine phosphate in providing ATP at the time of immediate demand during early phase of muscle exercise.

Creatinine is non-toxic excretory compound which is produced by spontaneous and irreversible dehydration of creatine during its metabolic turnover.

2% of total creatine is converted to creatinine which comes to plasma.

Amount of creatine and thus creatinine is directly proportional to the muscle mass of the individual which remains constant. Thus, creatinine is a better marker than urea for assessing the kidney function as the level of creatinine, unlike urea, does not change with dietary intake of protein.

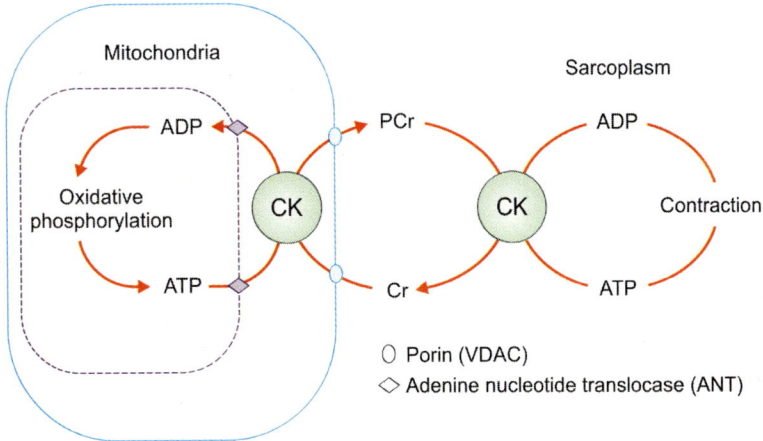

ADP: Adenosine diphosphate; CK: Creatinine kinase; PCr: Phosphocreatine; ATP: Adenosine triphosphate; Cr: Free creatinine

Fig. 9.1: Phosphocreatine as a source of ATP

Three factors determine the level of creatinine in the plasma:
1. Muscle mass
2. Rate of creatine turnover
3. Renal function

Serum creatinine is not a very sensitive marker for assessment of renal function as >50% deterioration in the renal function results in measurable increase of serum creatinine.

Following methods may be used for estimation of serum creatinine:
1. Chemical method: Jaffe's reaction
2. Enzymatic method: Creatininase

CHEMICAL METHOD

Jaffe's Reaction

It was devised by Jaffe in 1886.

Principle

It is a chemical method where creatinine is made to react with picric acid in alkaline medium to provide orange red-colored chromogen of creatinine picrate, which is quantified at 490 nm in colorimeter.

Reagents Required

For preparation of PFF:
1. H_2SO_4: 2/3 M
2. 10% sodium tungstate solution

For actual Jaffe reaction:
1. Saturated picric acid solution
2. 5% NaOH
3. Creatinine standard: 1 mg%

Procedure

Preparation of protein free filtrate (PFF) [test tube A]: 1 mL of DW + 1 mL of whole blood + 1 mL of sodium tungstate + 1 mL of H_2SO_4 is taken in a centrifuge tube (total 4 mL) and is mixed well. It is centrifuged at 3,000 rpm for 3 minutes, and supernatant is used for creatinine estimation which is free of protein (protein free filtrate).

Jaffe reaction:
- Three test tubes are taken and marked as B, S, T.
- Reagents are added as given in Table 9.1.

| Table 9.1: Scheme detail for creatinine quantification by Jaffe's method ||||
Reagents	B (blank) mL	S (standard) mL	T (test) mL
5% NaOH	1	1	1
Sat. picric acid	1	1	1
Creatinine standard (1 mg%)		1	
DW	4	3	2
PFF			2
Total	**6**	**6**	**6**

- Test tubes are shaken to mix the solution and they are placed at 37°C for 10 minutes. Thereafter, OD reading is taken at 520 nm (Fig. 9.2).

Calculation

Concentration of creatinine in serum = OD of test/OD of standard × amount of standard (in mg)/volume of serum (in mL) × 100

OD of test/OD of standard × 0.01/0.5 × 100

OD of test/OD of standard × 2

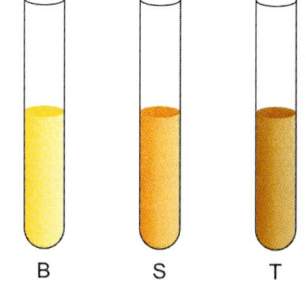

Fig. 9.2: Creatinine estimation by Jaffe's reaction

Interpretation

- Normal range of creatinine in healthy male is 0.9 to 1.3 mg/dL.
- Normal range of creatinine in healthy female is 0.6 to 1.1 mg/dL.

High creatinine: Seen in condition like renal failure.

Jaffe reaction is non-specific and false positive result is given by:
- Acetone
- Acetoacetic acid
- Cephalosporin
- Ascorbate
- Glucose
- Pyruvate

To increase the specificity of creatinine assessment, these methods of creatinine estimation may be adopted:
1. Kinetic Jaffe's method
2. Coupled enzymatic method
3. Isotope dilution mass spectrometry (IDMS)

Kinetic Jaffe's method: Here rate of change of absorbance is measured after adding the serum sample with alkaline picrate.

Coupled enzymatic method: Reaction with combination of various enzymes like creatininase, creatine phosphokinase, pyruvate kinase, LDH, etc. is used to quantify the creatinine.

Isotope dilution mass spectrometry (IDMS): It is reference method for assessment of serum creatinine.

Urinary Creatinine Estimation

As there is large amount of creatinine excreted in urine, urine needs to be diluted 100 times before the urinary creatinine is estimated, and the result is multiplied by 100.

Same method as adopted for serum creatinine assessment may be utilized for urinary creatinine assessment.

Calculation of creatinine clearance: Formula is

$$\text{Creatinine clearance} = \frac{UV}{P}$$

U = urinary creatinine level (mg/dL)

P = plasma creatinine level (mg/dL)
V = volume of urine in mL per minute [calculated as]

$$= \frac{\text{volume of urine in 24 hr collection (in mL)}}{24 \times 60}$$

(24 is the hours in a day and 60 is the minutes in an hour)

Estimation of Creatinine

Method Used: _____
_____
_____
_____

Observation

OD of test: _____

OD of standard: _____

Calculation

Concentration of creatinine in serum (mg/dL) =

OD of test/OD of standard × amount of standard/volume of serum × 100

Result

_____
_____
_____

Clinical Correlation: _____
_____
_____
_____

Dated: _____   **Teacher's Signature**

Clearance Study: _____
_____

U (Urinary creatinine in mg/dL): _____
_____

V (Volume of urine per minute): _____
_____

P (Plasma creatinine in mg/dL): _____
_____

Formula

$$\text{Creatinine clearance} = \frac{UV}{P}$$

Estimation of Creatinine in Serum and Other Biological Fluids

VIVA VOCE

Q1. What is the source of plasma creatinine?
Ans. Creatinine is produced after non-enzymatic spontaneous dehydration of creatine. Creatine is the compound which is stored in the muscle in the form of creatine phosphate (phosphagen). Creatine phosphate is the instant source of ATP and provides ATP during muscle exercise.

Q2. What are all factors that determine level of creatinine in the plasma?
Ans. Three factors that determine the level of creatinine in the plasma are:
a. Muscle mass
b. Rate of creatine turnover
c. Renal function

Q3. In what aspect, creatinine is a better marker of kidney function compared to urea?
Ans. Creatinine is a better marker than urea for assessing the kidney function as the level of creatinine, unlike urea, does not change with dietary intake of protein.

Q4. Whether the creatinine is sensitive marker for assessing renal dysfunction? If no, then why?
Ans. Serum creatinine is not a very sensitive marker for assessment of renal dysfunction as >50% deterioration in the renal function results in measurable increase of serum creatinine. In other words, to find out kidney dysfunction by altered creatinine value alone, considerable loss of kidney function should be underlying factor.

Q5. What all methods you know to estimate serum creatinine?
Ans. Following methods may be used for estimation of serum creatinine:
- *Chemical method*: Jaffe's reaction
- *Enzymatic method*: Creatininase

Q6. What is the principle of Jaffe's method of creatinine assessment?
Ans. Underlying principle of Jaffe's method is that, "When creatinine is made to react with picric acid in alkaline medium to provide orange red-colored chromogen of creatinine picrate, which is quantified at 490 nm in colorimeter. The amount of colored complex formed is directly proportional to the amount of creatinine in the biological fluid".

Q7. What wavelength will you measure the OD for alkaline picrate formed during Jaffe's reaction and why?
Ans. Optical density (OD) is the measure of absorbance and OD of alkaline picrate (which is orange red color complex) is taken at 520 nm.

This nm wavelength is selected because this is complimentary wavelength for orange red color complex and it shows maximum absorption.

Q8. What is the normal range of creatinine in male and female?
Ans.
- Normal range of creatinine in healthy male is 0.9 to 1.3 mg/dL
  - Normal range of creatinine in healthy female is 0.6 to 1.1 mg/dL.

Q9. What are the positive interferences in Jaffe's reaction? State any four compounds which give positive Jaffe's reaction.
Ans. Jaffe reaction is non-specific and false positive result is given by following compounds:
- Acetone
- Acetoacetic acid

- Cephalosporin
- Ascorbate
- Glucose
- Pyruvate

Q10. Whether Jaffe reaction is specific for creatinine?
Ans. No. Jaffe reaction is non-specific for creatinine and many other substances other than creatinine like acetoacetate, bilirubin, protein, etc. also give coloured complex resulting in higher estimation of creatinine in biological fluid.

Q11. How to increase the specificity of Jaffe reaction for creatinine estimation?
Ans. Kinetic method of Jaffe reaction gives more accurate result of creatinine in biological fluid compared to simple Jaffe reaction.

Q12. What is kinetic method of Jaffe reaction?
Ans. In this method, the reading is taken in window period of 20 to 80 seconds, as in this time period, it is the creatinine which interacts most with saturated picric acid used.

Acetoacetate is quick to act and it gives color before 20 second and proteins are slow to act which give color beyond 80 seconds.

This way kinetic method of Jaffe reaction is more specific for creatinine estimation.

CHAPTER 10

Estimation of Uric Acid in Serum

OVERVIEW OF URIC ACID AND ITS CLINICAL IMPORTANCE

Uric acid is chemically 2, 4, 6 trihydroxypurine.

Uric acid is the catabolic end product of purine nucleotide metabolism. Majority of uric acid in the body is originating from endogenous pool of purine nucleotides but significant amount of uric acid is also produced via catabolism of dietary nucleotides.

Major route of excretion of uric acid is kidney which removes approximately 10% of total uric acid 'filtered' through glomerulus. It is also important to be noted that kidney is responsible for elimination of 70% of total uric acid which is removed from the body, remainder is entering in GIT where they are degraded by intestinal enzyme.

Uric acid has dissociation constant (pKa) of 5.7, at pH above this (physiological pH = 7.4), uric acid remains in ionized form(urate/monosodium urate/MSU) which is sparingly soluble (but certainly more soluble than uric acid). If the concentration of MSU increases beyond 6.8 mg/dL, it tends to precipitate in joints and tissues. This results in a clinical condition known as gout which is characterized by painful joint swelling and deposition of tophi. Tophi are crystalline deposits of uric acid and urates. At lower pH (in acidosis), it remains in the form of uric acid which is insoluble and tends to form uric acid crystals.

Measurement of uric acid is useful in:
- Diagnosis and management of gout
- To monitor patients on chemotherapy
- To detect kidney dysfunction.

Following methods may be used for estimation of plasma uric acid:
1. Chemical method {phosphotungstic method (Caraway method)}
2. Coupled enzymatic method [uricase-peroxidase reaction]

Phosphotungstic Method (Caraway Method)

Principle

Uric acid is a reducing reagent which reduces phosphotungstic acid in alkaline media to convert it to tungsten blue, which is read at colorimeter at 650 nm (red filter).

Uric acid is oxidized in this reaction to allantoin which is produced as byproduct.

Protein free filtrate (PFF) is used because protein interfere with the test.

Estimation of Uric Acid in Serum

Reagents Required
1. Sodium carbonate (10%)
2. Tungstic acid reagent
3. Phosphotungstic acid
4. Uric acid standard (1 mg%)

Procedure

Step 1: Preparation of protein free filtrate (PFF) [test tube A]: 5.4 mL of tungstic acid reagent +0.6 mL of whole blood is taken in a centrifuge tube (total 6 mL) and is mixed well and kept for 10 minutes at room temperature. It is centrifuged at 3,000 rpm for 5 minutes, and supernatant is used for uric acid estimation which is free of protein (protein free filtrate).

Step 2: Three test tubes are taken and marked as B, S, T (Fig. 10.1).
Reagents are added as given in Table 10.1.

Test tubes are shaken to mix the solution and they are kept at room temperature (37°C) bath for 15 minutes. Thereafter they are cooled and OD reading is taken at 650 nm.

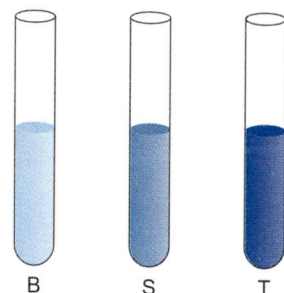

Fig. 10.1: Phosphotungstic method (Caraway method) of uric acid estimation

Table 10.1: Scheme detail for uric acid quantification by phosphotungstic method (Caraway method)			
Reagents	B (blank) mL	S (standard) mL	T (test) mL
Standard uric acid (1 mg%)		3	
PFF			3
DW	3		
Sodium carbonate	1	1	1
Phosphotungstic acid	1	1	1
Total	5	5	5

Calculation

Concentration of uric acid in serum = OD of test/OD of standard × amount of standard (in mg)/volume of serum (in mL) × 100

OD of test/OD of standard × 0.03/0.3 × 100

OD of test/OD of standard × 10

Coupled Enzymatic Method for Uric Acid Assessment

In this method, uricase acts on uric acid to convert it to allantoin, H_2O_2 is the byproduct in this reaction.

Rxn (Fig. 10.2)

H_2O_2 is next acted upon by peroxidase enzyme which converts it to H_2O and nascent oxygen [O].

Nascent oxygen [O] acts on indicator dye which is converted to colored complex. Color thus produced is directly proportional to the amount of uric acid and OD is measured colorimetrically then calculated for uric acid concentration.

Bilirubin and ascorbate act as negative interferences in this method as they readily destroy H_2O_2.

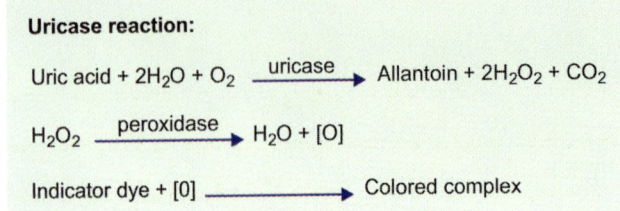

Fig. 10.2: Coupled enzymatic method for uric acid estimation

Interpretation

Normal range of uric acid in a healthy adult male: 3.6–7.2 mg/dL.
Normal range of uric acid in a healthy adult female: 2.6–6.0 mg/dL.

High uric acid: Seen in condition like:
- Gout
- Lesch-Nyhan syndrome
- PRPP synthetase mutation
- Von Gierke's disease
- Fructose intolerance
- Purine-rich diet
- Lactic acidosis
- Renal disease
- Chemotherapy for leukemia, lymphoma

Low uric acid
- Liver disorder
- Fanconi syndrome (defect in tubular reabsorption)
- Overenthusiastic treatment with allopurinol

Estimation of Uric Acid

Method Used: _____
_____
_____
_____

Observation

OD of test: _____

OD of standard: _____

Calculation

Concentration of uric acid in serum (mg/dL) =

OD of test/OD of standard × amount of standard/volume of serum × 100

Result

_____
_____
_____

Clinical Correlation: _____
_____
_____
_____

Dated: _____   **Teacher's Signature**

VIVA VOCE

Q1. What is the chemical nature of uric acid?
Ans. Uric acid is chemically 2, 4, 6 trihydroxypurine.

Q2. What is the source of uric acid?
Ans. Uric acid is the catabolic end product of purine nucleotide metabolism. Majority of it is produced by endogenous purine nucleotide metabolism though small amount is also produced by dietary purine nucleotide.

Q3. What is gout?
Ans. If the concentration of monosodium urate (MSU) increases beyond 6.8 mg/dL, it tends to precipitate in joints and tissues. This clinical condition is known as gout characterized by painful joint swelling and deposition of tophi.

Q4. What are tophi?
Ans. Tophi are crystalline deposits of uric acid and urates.

Q5. What is the characteristic feature of crystals which are deposited in gout?
Ans. Monosodium urate crystals which are deposited are negatively birefringent crystals.

Q6. Following methods may be used for estimation of plasma uric acid.
Ans.
1. Chemical method [phosphotungstic method (Caraway method)]
2. Coupled enzymatic method (uricase-peroxidase reaction)

Q7. What is the principle of phosphotungstic method (Caraway method)?
Ans. Uric acid is a reducing reagent which reduces phosphotungstic acid in alkaline media to convert it to tungsten blue. The amount of tungsten blue produced is directly proportional to the amount of uric acid. The color developed is read at colorimeter at 650 nm/red filter.

Q8. What is the normal range of uric acid in male and female?
Ans.
- Normal range of uric acid in a healthy adult male: 3.6–7.2 mg/dL.
- Normal range of uric acid in a healthy adult female: 2.6–6.0 mg/dL.

Q9. Mention a few conditions when the level of uric acid will be high?
Ans. Conditions where uric acid level will be high (hyperuricemia) are:
- Gout
- Lesch-Nyhan syndrome
- PRPP synthetase mutation
- Von Gierke's disease
- Fructose intolerance
- Purine-rich diet like excess consumption of mushroom, cauliflower, spinach, meat, etc.
- Lactic acidosis
- Renal disease
- Chemotherapy for leukemia, lymphoma

Q10. How alcohol consumption precipitates gout attack?
Ans. Alcohol metabolism increases level of NADH which tends to convert pyruvate to lactate resulting in lactic acidosis. Excretion of uric acid is impaired in lactic acidosis resulting in hyperuricemia and gout.

Q11. What is the difference in primary and secondary gout?
Ans. When the hyperuricemia and gout is because of defect in purine nucleotide metabolism it is known as primary gout and if the hyperuricemia and gout is associated with other diseases like carbohydrate metabolism defect (Von Gierke disease, fructose intolerance, galactosemia, etc.) or any other defect, it is called secondary gout.

Notes

CHAPTER

11

Liver Function Test: An Overview

Competency

Bi 6.14 [A to D]: Describe the tests that are commonly done in clinical practice to assess the functions of these organs (kidney, liver, thyroid and adrenal glands)

All the tests which are being done to assess the liver function are collectively known as liver function test (LFT).

Two important points to be noticed regarding LFT are:

1. LFT is a misnomer, as all the tests done under this heading do not necessarily assess the liver function. For example, enzyme assays (AST, ALT, ALP) done under LFT, rather denote the extent of damage of hepatocyte (in other words, the dysfunction of hepatocyte) (Table 11.1).

Table 11.1: Tests which are done under LFT to assess diverse roles of liver	
1. Serum bilirubin (total and conjugated)	To assess the liver dysfunction
2. Total protein and serum albumin, A:G ratio	
3. Prothrombin time	

4. Urine: Bile pigment
       Bile salt
       Urobilinogen	

5. AST (SGOT)*	To assess liver cell damage
6. ALT (SGPT)*	
7. Alkaline phosphatase (ALP)	
8. γ-glutamyltransferase (GGT)	

*Relative increase of ALT and AST hints towards type of cell damage. ALT is confined to cytosol and AST is within mitochondrial matrix of hepatocyte. If ALT increases more than AST, it indicates plasma membrane damage (inflammatory or infective condition). On the other hand, if AST is increased more than ALT, it indicates mitochondrial membrane damage in addition to plasma membrane damage (infiltrative disorder).

Liver Function Test: An Overview

Normal range of various parameters being assessed in LFT:
- Total bilirubin: 0.2–1.0 mg/dL
- Unconjugated bilirubin (indirect): 0.2–0.7 mg/dL
- Conjugated bilirubin (direct): 0.1–0.4 mg/dL
- AST: 5–30 U/L
- ALT: 5–40 U/L
- ALP: 30–120 IU/L
- GGT: 5–30 IU/L
- Prothrombin time: 11–15 sec
- Total protein: 6 to 8 g/dL
- Albumin: 3.5 to 5.5 g/dL

2. Because of large reserve capacity of liver, test done to assess impairment of metabolic function (synthetic and excretory) of the liver, e.g. albumin level, clotting factor assessment (prothrombin test), bilirubin level assessment, is relatively an insensitive indicator of liver disease.

All the tests being done under LFT which assess liver dysfunction, evaluate disease severity, monitor therapy and assess prognosis are given in Table 11.2.

Table 11.2: Blood test	
To check for excretory function of liver	1. Serum total bilirubin
To differentiate between hepatitis and obstructive jaundice	2. Serum conjugated bilirubin
	3. Serum unconjugated bilirubin
To check for hepatocellular damage	4. AST (aspartate transaminase)
	5. ALT (alanine transaminase)
To check for cholestasis	6. ALP (alkaline phosphatase)
To check for obstructive lesions	7. γGT (gamma-glutamyl transferase)
To check for synthetic function	8. Total protein
	9. Serum albumin
	10. Serum globulins
	11. Prothrombin time
To assess excretory function of liver	12. Blood ammonia level

Enzyme Marker of Liver Disease

Plasma aminotransferase (AST and ALT), ALP and gamma-glutamyl transferase (GGT) are important tests which differentiate hepatocellular disease from cholestatic disease.

AST (Aspartate Transaminase)

AST is distributed in high concentration in heart muscle, skeletal muscle, kidney and RBC. Raised plasma AST level hence is non-specific to liver disease and may be elevated in following conditions:
1. Liver disease:
   - Cirrhosis
   - Cholestatic jaundice
   - Malignant infiltration of liver

- Acute viral hepatitis
- Toxic hepatitis
2. Myocardial infarction
3. Skeletal muscle disease
4. Hemolysis
5. Trauma or surgery
6. Circulatory failure with shock and hypoxia

ALT (Alanine Transaminase)

ALT is distributed in liver and to lesser extent in skeletal muscle, kidney and heart.
Raised ALT in plasma is rather more specific to liver disease compared to AST.
In following conditions, plasma ALT will be raised:
1. Circulatory failure with shock and hypoxia
2. Acute viral hepatitis
3. Toxic hepatitis
4. Cirrhosis
5. Congestive cardiac failure
6. Cholestatic jaundice
7. Surgery or trauma

ALP (Alkaline Phosphatase)

ALP is ectoenzyme distributed at small intestine mucosa, proximal convoluted tubule of kidney, osteoblast of bone, liver and placenta. Zinc is a constituent metal ion for ALP and Mg^{++}, Mn^{++} and Co^{++} are activator of enzyme. ALP synthesis by hepatocyte is induced in response to any biliary tract obstruction (stone, malignancy head of pancreas). Level of ALP may increase 10 to 12-fold in case of obstruction of biliary tract.

Various isoenzymes of ALP can be separated by electrophoresis. Liver ALP moves maximally towards anode.

γGT (Gamma-Glutamyl Transpeptidase or Gamma-Glutamyl Transferase)

γGT is present in microsome. It is found at proximal convoluted tubule, liver, pancreas and GIT. Though the enzyme is most abundant in PCT, the serum enzyme predominantly comes from liver. Unlike ALP, γGT is not increased in bone disease. So γGT estimation is useful to differentiate liver disease from bone disease in case of elevated ALP.

γGT is elevated manyfold in alcoholic liver disease.

If the elevation is primarily of aminotransferases, then hepatocellular disease is likely; and if elevation is primarily of alkaline phosphatase (ALP), then cholestatic disorder (obstructive disorder) is likely.

To confirm the hepatobiliary origin of raised ALP, simultaneous assessment of γGT (γ-glutamyl transferase) should be done, which parallels the level of ALP in case GGT is of hepatobiliary origin.

- ALT is purely cytosolic and AST is both cytosolic and mitochondrial.
- AST is widely distributed in heart, liver, skeletal muscle and kidney while ALT is distributed in liver and kidney.
- Assessment of ALT is more specific for liver disorder compared to AST.

Tests to Assess the Synthetic Function of Liver

Various tests to be done to assess the synthetic function of liver are described below.

Albumin: As the liver is responsible for synthesis of albumin, estimation of serum albumin is important marker of liver synthetic capacity.

Prothrombin time: Liver is responsible for formation of clotting factors (except factor V). Hence, prothrombin time gives a fair idea regarding liver functional capacity.

Blood ammonia level: It is raised, if liver is not able to detoxify ammonia and convert it to urea.

Urine Investigations to Assess Liver Function

Urine investigations to be done to assess liver function are described below.

Traditional methods of assessment of urinary bilirubin, bile salt, and urobilinogen are commonly used in day-to-day practice.

1. **Fouchet's test** [for detection of bilirubin in urine]: Conjugated bilirubin is raised in blood in cases of obstructive jaundice and also in hepatic jaundice. Only conjugated bilirubin being water soluble gets excreted in urine. Unconjugated bilirubin on the other hand being water insoluble does not come out in the urine. Bilirubin in the urine is detected by 'Fouchet's test' which gives green color when positive. Hence, positive Fouchet's test suggests presence of conjugated bilirubin in the urine and hence obstructive juandice or obstructive stage of hepatic juandice.
2. **Hay's sulfur test:** This test detects presence of bile salts in urine, which is excreted in case of obstructive jaundice. Bile salt reduces surface tension and when sulfur powder is sprinkled on the surface of urine in a test tube, sulfur powder sinks at the bottom of the tube. This denotes presence of bile salt in the urine and hence obstructive jaundice.
3. **Ehrlich test:** This test detects urobilinogen (UBG) in the urine. UBG is produced in GIT lumen from bilirubin and enters in enterohepatic circulation, so in obstructive jaundice, when bile is not reaching the duodenum, UBG is not formed and urine is tested negative for UBG. [Negative Ehrlich test denotes obstructive jaundice.]

To check for bilirubin and urobilinogen in the urine, reagent strips are also available.

For urinary bilirubin, 'Ictostix' is used. It includes diazotized 2, 4-dichloraniline which reacts with bilirubin and produces azobilirubin. "Chlorpromazine" gives false positive result.

For urinary urobilinogen, 'Urobilistix' is used. It includes 'para-dimethylaminobenzaldehyde' which reacts with urobilinogen. Para-aminosalicylic acid and some sulphonamides give false positive result.

Marked presence of urinary urobilinogen and lack of bilirubin in the urine suggest hemolytic jaundice.

Finding in blood, urine and stool in different types of jaundice is summarized in Table 11.3.

Assessment of Serum Bilirubin [Total and Conjugated]
The basic principle behind assessment of serum bilirubin is 'Van den Bergh reaction'.

Van den Bergh Test
In this, bilirubin reacts with diazotized sulfanilic acid to produce azobilirubin which is purple in color. It can assess both conjugated and unconjugated bilirubins in direct and indirect reaction, respectively. Conjugated bilrubin is water soluble and hence it gives Van den Bergh reaction in aqueous medium itself **(direct reaction)**.

Unconjugated bilirubin gets solubilized after addition of methyl alcohol and starts giving Van den Bergh reaction **(indirect reaction)**.

Table 11.3: Findings in blood, urine and stool in different types of jaundice			
	Prehepatic	*Hepatic*	*Post-hepatic*
Color of stool	Dark color (due to stercobilinogen)	Normal	Clay/pale stool
Bile pigment (bilirubin)	–	±	++
Urinary finding (bile salt)	–	±	++
Urobilinogen (UBG)	++ (Due to increased urobilinogen)	+	–
Finding in blood			
T. bilirubin	↑↑	↑↑	↑↑
Conjugated bilirubin	↑	↑↑	↑↑↑
Unconjugated bilirubin	↑↑↑	↑↑	↑
ALP	–	↑	↑
γGT	–	–	↑

So, the color is read before and after the addition of methyl alcohol in the reaction mixture which gives "conjugated bilirubin" and "total bilirubin" estimation, respectively. To find out the unconjugated bilirubin fraction, conjugated bilirubin value is deducted from total bilirubin value.

In hemolytic jaundice, unconjugated bilirubin is raised in plasma, because production of bilirubin is more than the capacity of liver to conjugate and excrete it, raising the level of unconjugated bilirubin.

In post-hepatic (obstructive) jaundice, it is conjugated bilirubin which is effluxed in blood circulation because of obstruction in the passage of conjugated bilirubin towards intestinal lumen.

In hepatic jaundice, both unconjugated and conjugated bilirubins are raised in the plasma. It is due to impaired hepatic functioning which raises unconjugated form and intrahepatic cholestasis due to edematous hepatic cell which results in raised conjugated bilirubin.

Diazotized sulphanilic acid + Bilirubin → Azobilirubin (purple)

In nutshell: Van den Bergh test

Direct test: Given by conjugated bilirubin. It is positive in obstructive jaundice when level of conjugated bilirubin increases.

Indirect test: Given by unconjugated bilirubin. Here Van den Bergh test gives positive result only after addition of alcohol and hence it is called indirect test and unconjugated bilirubin is known as indirect bilirubin. In hemolytic anemia, unconjugated bilirubin increases, which gives indirect test +ve.

Biphasic: When serum has increased conjugated and unconjugated bilirubins (as seen in hepatic disease) the Van den Bergh reaction is biphasic which means that purple color is produced immediately which gets intensified on adding the alcohol.

Notes

CHAPTER

12

Estimation of Bilirubin

Competency

BI 11.12: Demonstrate the estimation of serum bilirubin.

Bilirubin is derived from heme during its catabolism. Heme is acted upon by heme oxygenase enzyme which converts it to biliverdin which is a green pigment. Biliverdin is reduced to bilirubin by biliverdin reductase to produce bilirubin which is the orangish yellow pigment (Fig. 12.1).

Rxn

Per day 250–300 mg of bilirubin is produced which should be excreted from the body. Out of this amount of bilirubin, majority of bilirubin (85%) is produced from old RBCs and lesser amount (15%) is produced from ineffective erythropoiesis in the bone marrow. Catabolism of other heme protein like catalase, peroxidase, myoglobin, various cytochromes, etc. also contribute to this minor fraction of bilirubin.

Bilirubin thus produced in reticuloendothelial cells are unconjugated which is not soluble in the plasma, hence it binds with albumin for transportation purpose. Liver uptakes this bilirubin, leaving behind albumin and conjugates it with glucuronic acid in presence of enzyme **UDP**

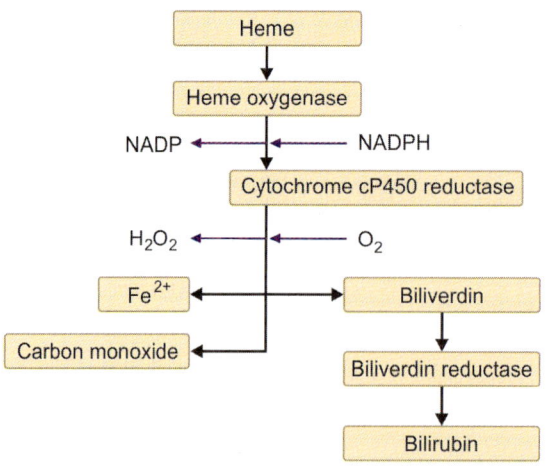

Fig. 12.1: Heme degradation and synthesis of bilirubin

glucuronyl transferase. Bilirubin monoglucuronide and bilirubin diglucuronides are thus produced which are excreted in the intestine via bile.

Any interruption in conjugation or excretion of this conjugated bilirubin results in abnormal accumulation of bilirubin in the body, a **condition known as jaundice**.

HISTORY OF BILIRUBIN ANALYSIS

- **Ehrlich** in 1883 first described a method by which urinary bilirubin makes a coloured complex with diazotized sulfanilic acid. This was classically known as **'Diazo reaction'**.
- In 1913, **Van den Bergh** proposed a method where Diazo reaction could be applied for serum sample as well, in presence of an **accelerator**.
- In 1937, **Malloy and Evelyn** proposed a method where **50% methanol** was used as an accelerator for quantification of plasma bilirubin.
- Followed by this, in year 1938, **Jendrassik and Grof** proposed a method in which plasma bilirubin was quantitated using **caffeine-benzoate-acetate as an accelerator**.
- Nowadays most of the methods of estimation of bilirubin are based on Malloy and Evelyn method, in spite of the fact that the **Jendrassik and Grof method is considered as candidate reference method by AACC (American Association of Clinical Chemistry)**.

Malloy and Evelyn Method

Principle

This method is based on the principle of Van den Bergh, where plasma or serum bilirubin interacts with diazotized sulfanilic acid to form azobilirubin which is reddish purple compound and the color thus produced is directly proportional to amount of soluble bilirubin and it is measured colorimetrically at 560 nm.

Test is done twice, first before addition of an accelerator and second after addition of an accelerator. Methanol is the accelerator used in this method.

The measurement in the first test (before addition of an accelerator) measures only conjugated bilirubin which is polar and soluble.

The measurement in the second test (after addition of an accelerator) measures total bilirubin (conjugated + unconjugated). This is due to conversion of unconjugated bilirubin to soluble and hence measurable form after addition of an accelerator (methanol).

Reagents Required

1. Diazo reagent (sulfanilic acid and sodium nitrate in HCl)
2. Diazo blank: 1.5% HCl
3. Methanol
4. **Bilirubin standard:** 280 mg/dL of methyl red is used as a standard. It gives optical density of 0.32 which is equivalent of 8 mg% of bilirubin concentration.

Actual bilirubin powder is not used to make the standard, reason being bilirubin is a photolabile compound and it deteriorates on exposure to day light. This standard when used, there is high possibility of getting erratic result, hence artificial standard of methyl red is used.

Procedure

Three test tubes are taken and marked as T1, T2 and control (C). Reagents are added in these tubes according to Table 12.1.

All test tubes are shaken well to mix the content. Kept in dark for 30 min. OD is read at 560 nm.

Table 12.1: Scheme detail for bilirubin quantification (both conjugated and total) by Malloy and Evelyn method

Reagents	T1 mL (for total bil)	T2 mL (for conjugated bil)	Control (mL)
Diazo reagent	0.5	0.5	
Diazo blank			0.5
Serum	0.2	0.2	0.2
Methanol	2.5		2.5
DW	1.8	4.3	1.8
Total	5	5	5

Calculation

- Concentration of total bilirubin in serum = OD of test (T1)–OD of control/OD of standard × 8
- Concentration of conjugated bilirubin in serum = OD of test (T2)–OD of control/OD of standard × 8 [OD of standard is 0.32]
- Concentration of unconjugated bilirubin = total bilirubin–conjugated bilirubin

Interpretation

- Normal value of total bilirubin: 0.2 to 1.2 mg/dL.
- Normal value of conjugated bilirubin: 0.0 to 0.2 mg/dL.
- Normal value of unconjugated bilirubin: 0.2 to 1.0 mg/dL.

Estimation of Serum Bilirubin

Method Used: _____
_____
_____
_____

Observation

OD of T1: _____

OD of T2: _____

OD of Standard: _____

Calculation

Total bilirubin (mg/dL) =

OD of T1–OD of control/OD of standard × Amount of standard/Volume of serum × 100

Conjugated bilirubin (mg/dL) =

OD of T2–OD of control/OD of standard × Amount of standard/Volume of serum × 100

Unconjugated bilirubin (mg/dL) = Total bilirubin–Conjugated bilirubin

Result

Total bilirubin =
Conjugated bilirubin =
Unconjugated bilirubin =

Clinical Correlation: _____
_____
_____
_____

Dated: _____   **Teacher's Signature**

VIVA VOCE

Q1. What is the source of bilirubin and how is it produced?
Ans. Heme degradation produces bilirubin.
Following are the steps: Figure 12.1.

Q2. How many types actually constitute total bilirubin?
Ans. There are three types of bilirubin which constitute total bilirubin:
  i. Conjugated bilirubin
  ii. Unconjugated bilirubin
  iii. Delta bilirubin (conjugated bilirubin bound with albumin)

Q3. What is the normal level of various types of bilirubin?
Ans.
- Normal value of total bilirubin: 0.2 to 1.2 mg/dL.
- Normal value of conjugated bilirubin: 0.0 to 0.2 mg/dL.
- Normal value of unconjugated bilirubin: 0.2 to 1.0 mg/dL.

Q4. What is the transport protein for transportation of unconjugated bilirubin?
Ans. Albumin

Q5. What is jaundice?
Ans. Any interruption in conjugation or excretion of this conjugated bilirubin results in abnormal accumulation of bilirubin in the body, a condition known as jaundice.

Level of bilirubin >2 mg/dL results in clinical juandice and bilirubin level 1.0 to 2.0 mg/dL results in latent juandice.

Q6. How many types of jaundice you know?
Ans.
- Pre-hepatic (hemolytic)
- Hepatic
- Post-hepatic (obstructive)

Q7. What is the role of addition of methanol in Van den Bergh method of bilirubin assessment?
Ans. Methanol is said to be an accelerator in this and it converts unconjugated bilirubin to conjugated bilirubin. So, before addition of ethanol, only conjugated bilirubin is estimated but after addition of methanol the total bilirubin is estimated.

Notes

CHAPTER 13

Estimation of AST/SGOT

> **Competency**
>
> **BI 2.2:** Observe the estimation of SGOT.

AST (aspartate aminotransferase) is the transaminase belonging to class II (transferase) of enzyme classification. This enzyme was previously known as SGOT (serum glutamate oxaloacetate transaminase). This enzyme catalyses following transamination reaction and is dependent of pyridoxal phosphate (PLP) (Fig. 13.1).

$$\text{L-Aspartate} + \alpha\text{-ketoglutarate} \xrightarrow[\text{PLP}]{\text{AST}} \text{Oxaloacetate} + \text{L-Glutamate}$$

Fig. 13.1: Reaction catalyzed by AST

AST is widely distributed. Predominant organs where AST is found are the cardiac tissue, liver and skeletal muscle. Kidney, RBC, pancreas are other tissues where minor amount of this enzyme is found. In cells, AST is both cytosolic and mitochondrial. Normally, in the plasma, cytosolic fraction is found, but in case of cell necrosis, it is mitochondrial fraction which predominantly is elevated.

Clinically, AST is evaluated to assess liver and skeletal muscle dysfunction. Even in cases of acute myocardial infarction (AMI), AST is quick to rise and last for long (rises within 6 hours of AMI, peaks at 24 hours, and return to baseline by 5 days).

In viral hepatitis, the level of AST may go up to more than 100 times of ULN (upper limit of normal), but in cirrhosis, the elevation is lesser (4 times of ULN).

Macro-AST: AST bound with anti-AST autoantibody produces macro-AST which has longer plasma half-life and results in persistent elevation of AST level even after recovery (up to tenfold of normal value).

Assessment of AST Level in the Plasma

Method Used

AST can be estimated by colorimetric method using 2, 4-dinitrophenylhydrazine (Mohun and Cook 1957).

Principle

AST catalyses transamination of L-aspartate and alpha ketoglutarate to produce oxaloacetate (OAA) and glutamate. This reaction requires enzyme AST in presence of cofactor PLP (pyridoxal phosphate) (Fig. 13.2).

OAA then interacts with 2, 4-dinitrophenylhydrazine in alkaline medium to produce hydrazine which is reddish brown in color and is read at 520 nm (green filter). The intensity of color is proportional to the amount of ketoacid (OAA) present, which in turn is directly proportional to the amount of serum aspartate transaminase.

Thus, the measurement of OD (optical density) of colored solution gives the estimate of AST present in the serum.

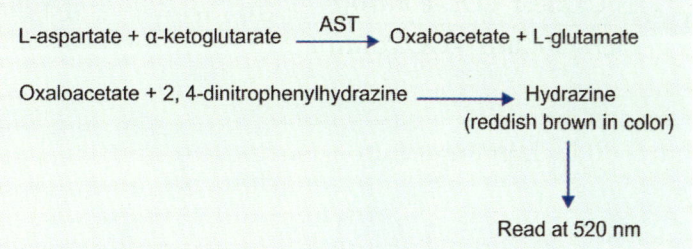

Fig. 13.2: Principle of AST assessment

Reagents Required

1. 0.1 M phosphate buffer (pH 7.4)
2. 2, 4-Dinitrophenylhydrazine (DNPH): 1 mM
3. NaOH (0.4 N)
4. *Substrate*: Consists of L-aspartate and alpha-ketoglutarate in phosphate buffer. 0.30 gram of L-aspartic acid and 50 mg of alpha-ketoglutarate are dissolved in 20 mL of phosphate buffer. 1.1 mL of 10% NaOH is added to bring the pH to 7.5. Further the volume is adjusted to 100 mL with addition of phosphate buffer.
5. *Standard*: Oxaloacetate solution (2 micromol/mL).

Assay Procedure

Four test tubes are taken and marked as T, S, C, B. Reagents are added in these test tubes as per plan in Table 13.1.

Read the OD of control, standard and test at 520 nm (green filter) after adjusting zero with blank.

Table 13.1: Scheme for estimation of AST by 2, 4-dinitrophenylhydrazine (Mohunand Cook) method				
Reagents	Test	Standard	Control	Blank
Substrate	1 mL	–	1 mL	–
Incubate at 37°C for 5 min				
Serum	0.2 mL	–	–	–
Incubate at 37°C for one hour				
DNPH reagent	1 mL	1 mL	1 mL	1 mL
Standard OAA solution	–	0.2 mL	–	–
Serum	–	–	0.2 ml	–
Mix and incubate at 37°C for 20 min				
NaOH	10 mL	10 mL	10 mL	10 mL
Mix and incubate at room temperature for 10 min				

Calculation

Use following formula to calculate the level of AST in serum (in IU/L)

$$\text{Serum level of AST} = \frac{\text{OD test} - \text{OD control}}{\text{OD standard} - \text{OD control}} \times \frac{\text{Amount of standard (mmol)}}{\text{Volume of serum (mL)}} \times 1000 \times \frac{1}{\text{Incubation time}}$$

$$\text{Serum level of AST} = \frac{\text{OD test} - \text{OD control}}{\text{OD standard} - \text{OD control}} \times \frac{0.4}{0.2} \times 1000 \times \frac{1}{60}$$

$$\text{Serum level of AST} = \frac{\text{OD test} - \text{OD control}}{\text{OD standard} - \text{OD control}} \times 33.3 \text{ IU/L}$$

Interpretation

Normal range: In adult: 5–30 U/L in the serum

Elevated in:
- Infective liver disorder
- Liver cirrhosis
- AMI (acute myocardial infarction)
- Skeletal muscle dystrophy

AST: ALT ratio (De Ritis ratio):
- The aspartate aminotransferase (AST) and alanine aminotransferase (ALT) ratio is known as De Ritis ratio (AAR). Normal ratio of AST and ALT is 1.15.
- Ratio >2 (3:1 or 4:1) denotes alcoholic liver disease.
- Ratio <1 denotes viral hepatitis and extrahepatic biliary obstruction.

Estimation of Serum AST

Method Used: _____
_____
_____
_____

Observation

OD of test: _____

OD of standard: _____

OD of control: _____

Calculation

_____
_____
_____

Result

_____
_____
_____

Clinical Correlation: _____
_____
_____
_____

Dated: _____   **Teacher's Signature**

VIVA VOCE

Q1. What is the full form of AST?

Ans. Aspartate transaminase

Q2. What is the other name of AST?

Ans. SGOT (serum glutamate oxaloacetate transaminase)

Q3. Is the AST elevation specific for liver damge?

Ans. No. AST is non-specific enzyme which is elevated in cardiac muscle damage also.

Q4. What is De Ritis ratio?

Ans. The aspartate aminotransferase (AST) and alanine aminotransferase (ALT) ratio is known as De Ritis ratio (AAR). Normal ratio of AST and ALT is 1.15.

Ratio >2 (3:1 or 4:1) denotes alcoholic liver disease.

Ratio <1 denotes viral hepatitis and extrahepatic biliary obstruction.

Notes

CHAPTER

14

Estimation of SGPT (ALT)

Competency
BI 2.2: Observe the estimation of SGPT.

CLINICAL OVERVIEW OF ALT

Alanine transaminase (ALT) is the transaminase belonging to class II (transferase) of enzyme classification. This enzyme was previously known as SGPT (serum glutamate pyruvate transaminase). This enzyme catalyses following transamination reaction and is dependent of pyridoxal phosphate (PLP).

$$\text{L-alanine} + \alpha\text{-ketoglutarate} \xrightarrow[\text{PLP}]{\text{ALT}} \text{Pyruvate} + \text{L-glutamate}$$

Fig. 14.1: Transamination catalysed by ALT

Though ALT is widely distributed like AST, ALT is considered more specific enzyme for the liver disease as compare to AST.

Clinically, assessment of ALT is limited to evaluation of liver disorder alone. It is elevated more than AST in inflammatory liver disorder and remains high for longer duration compared to AST.

Assessment of ALT Level in the Plasma

Method Used

ALT can be estimated by colorimetric method using 2, 4-dinitrophenylhydrazine (DNPH).

Principle

ALT catalyses transamination of L-alanine and alpha-ketoglutarate to produce pyruvate and L-glutamate. This reaction requires enzyme ALT in presence of cofactor PLP (pyridoxal phosphate).

Pyruvate then interacts with 2, 4-dinitrophenylhydrazine in alkaline medium to produce hydrazine which is reddish brown in color and is read at 520 nm (green filter). The intensity of color is proportional to the amount of ketoacid (pyruvate) present, which in turn is directly proportional to the amount of serum alanine transaminase (Fig. 14.2).

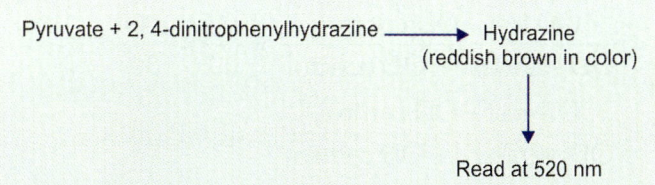

Fig. 14.2: Formation of colored product by pyruvate and DNPH interaction

Thus, the measurement of OD (optical density) of colored solution gives the estimate of ALT present in the serum.

Reagents Required

1. 0.1 M phosphate buffer (pH 7.4)
2. 2, 4-Dinitrophenylhydrazine (DNPH): 1 mM
3. NaOH (0.4 N)
4. Substrate: Consist of L-alanine and alpha-ketoglutarate in phosphate buffer. 5 grams of L-alanine and 20 mg of alpha-ketoglutarate are dissolved in 20 mL of phosphate buffer. 1.1 mL of 10% NaOH is added to bring the pH to 7.5. Further the volume is adjusted to 100 mL with addition of phosphate buffer.
5. Standard: Pyruvic acid solution (2 micro-mol/mL)

Assay Procedure

Four test tubes are taken and marked as T, S, C, B. Reagents are added in these test tubes as per plan in Table 14.1.

Read the OD of control, standard and test at 520 nm (green filter) after adjusting zero with blank.

Table 14.1: Scheme for estimation of ALT by 2, 4-dinitrophenylhydrazine (Mohunand Cook) method

Reagents	Test	Standard	Control	Blank
Substrate	1 mL	–	1 mL	–
Incubate at 37°C for 5 min				
Serum	0.2 mL	–	–	–
Incubate at 37°C for 30 min				
DNPH reagent	1 mL	1 mL	1 mL	1 mL
Standard pyruvate solution	–	0.2 mL	–	–
serum	–	–	0.2 ml	–
Mix and incubate at 37°C for 20 min				
NaOH	10 mL	10 mL	10 mL	10 mL
Mix and incubate at room temperature for 10 min				

Calculation

Use following formula to calculate the level of ALT in serum (in IU/L)

$$\text{Serum level of ALT} = \frac{\text{OD test} - \text{OD control}}{\text{OD standard} - \text{OD control}} \times \frac{\text{Amount of standard (mmol)}}{\text{Volume of serum (mL)}} \times \frac{100}{30} \times 1$$

$$\text{Serum level of ALT} = \frac{\text{OD test} - \text{OD control}}{\text{OD standard} - \text{OD control}} \times \frac{0.4}{0.2} \times \frac{1000}{30} \times 1$$

$$\text{Serum level of ALT} = \frac{\text{OD test} - \text{OD control}}{\text{OD standard} - \text{OD control}} \times 66.6 \text{ IU/L}$$

Interpretation

Normal range: In adult: 5–40 U/L in the serum.

Elevated in:
- Infective liver disorder
- Liver cirrhosis

AST: ALT ratio (De Ritis ratio):
- The aspartate aminotransferase (AST) and alanine aminotransferase (ALT) ratio is known as De Ritis ratio (AAR). Normal ratio of AST and ALT is 1.15.
- Ratio >2 (3:1 or 4:1) denotes alcoholic liver disease.
- Ratio <1 denotes viral hepatitis and extrahepatic biliary obstruction.

Estimation of Serum ALT

Method Used: _____
_____
_____
_____

Observation

OD of test: _____

OD of standard: _____

OD of control: _____

Calculation

_____
_____
_____

Result

_____
_____
_____

Clinical Correlation: _____
_____
_____
_____

Dated: _____ **Teacher's Signature**

VIVA VOCE

Q1. What is the full form of ALT?
Ans. Alanine transaminase

Q2. What is the other name of ALT?
Ans. SGPT (serum glutamate pyruvate transaminase)

Q3. Is the ALT elevation is specific for liver damge?
Ans. Yes.

Q4. What is De Ritis ratio?
Ans. The aspartate aminotransferase (AST) and alanine aminotransferase (ALT) ratio is known as De Ritis ratio (AAR). Normal ratio of AST and ALT is 1.15.

Ratio >2 (3:1 or 4:1) denotes alcoholic liver disease.

Ratio <1 denotes viral hepatitis and extrahepatic biliary obstruction.

Notes

CHAPTER

15

Estimation of ALP

Competency

BI 11.14: Demonstrate the estimation of alkaline phosphatase.

Alkaline phosphatase is the enzyme which hydrolyses various phosphate monoester under alkaline pH. (Optimum pH is 10.) It is found at cell surface of variety of tissues like liver, bone, placenta, intestine, kidney, spleen, etc.

Elevation of ALP is diagnostically useful in assessment of hepatobiliary disorder (both hepatic and obstructive conditions) and also bone disorders (especially those involving osteoblasts).

There are many isoenzymes of ALP: Liver, bone, intestine and placenta.

These isoenzymes can be separated by electrophoresis. Liver isoenzyme moves the fastest and the intestinal fraction moves the slowest.

Placental ALP is the most heat stable (resist heat at 65°C for 30 min) and bone ALP is the most heat labile.

Regan isoenzyme is special isoenzyme which is seen in 3 to 15% of cancer patients and is referred as **carcinoplacental alkaline phosphatase**. This isoenzyme is very similar to placental isoenzyme and shows similar heat stability. Regan isoenzyme is not useful in diagnosis of malignancy because of its appearance in a smaller number of cases, but its assessment is useful in knowing the response to therapy.

Assessment of Alkaline Phosphatase Enzyme
Method Used
1. King and Armstrong
2. Bowers and McComb

The method by King and Armstrong is described below.

Principle
Disodium phenylphosphate is acted upon by ALP to release phenol and sodium phosphate.

Released phenol then interacts with 4-aminoantipyrine (indicator dye) in presence of potassium ferricyanide and gives purple-colored complex which is read colorimetrically at 525 nm (green filter).

Estimation of ALP

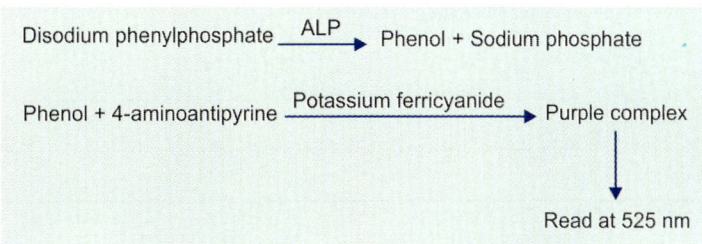

Fig. 15.1: Principle of ALP assessment

Reagents Required

1. 4-aminoantipyrine: 0.6%
2. Potassium ferricyanide: 2.4%
3. Disodium phenylphosphate: 0.01 M
4. Bicarbonate buffer of pH 10: 0.1 M
5. Buffered substrate
6. Phenol standard: 1 mg/dL

Assay Procedure

Four test tubes are taken and marked as T, S, B, C. Reagents are added in these test tubes as per plan in Table 15.1.

Mix well and read the color immediately at 525 nm (green filter).

Table 15.1: Scheme for estimation of ALP by King and Armstrong method				
Reagents	Test (mL)	Standard (mL)	Blank (mL)	Control (mL)
Bicarbonate buffer	1	1.1	1.1	1
Buffered substrate	1	1		1
Serum	0.1			
DW			1	
Incubate above for 15 min at 37°C				
Serum				0.1
NaOH (0.5 N)	0.8	0.8	0.8	0.8
Na$_2$CO$_3$	1.2	1.2	1.2	1.2
4-aminoantipyrine	1	1	1	1
Potassium ferricyanide	1	1	1	1

Calculation

Concentration of ALP in serum (KA units/dL) =
OD of test–OD of control/OD of standard–OD of blank × amount of standard/volume of serum × 100
OD of test–OD of control/OD of standard–OD of blank × 100 µg/0.1 × 100
OD of test–OD of control/OD of standard–OD of blank × 10

Estimation of Alkaline Phosphatase (ALP)

Method Used: _____
_____
_____
_____

Observation

OD of test: _____

OD of standard: _____

OD of blank: _____

OD of control: _____

Calculation

Concentration of ALP in serum (KA units /dL) =

OD of test–OD of control/OD of standard–OD of blank × amount of standard/volume of serum × 100

OD of test–OD of control/OD of standard–OD of blank × 100 µg/0.1 × 100

OD of test–OD of control/OD of standard–OD of blank × 10

Result

_____
_____
_____

Clinical Correlation: _____
_____
_____
_____

Dated: _____   **Teacher's Signature**

VIVA VOCE

Q1. What is the normal value of ALP in an adult male?
Ans. Normal value of ALP in an adult male is 30–120 IU/L.

Q2. How many isoenzymes are there in ALP?
Ans. There are many isoenzymes of ALP: Liver, bone, intestine and placenta.

Q3. How the isoenzymes can be separated?
Ans. These isoenzymes can be separated by electrophoresis.

Q4. Which isoenzyme moves the fastest and which moves the slowest on electrophoresis?
Ans. Liver isoenzyme moves the fastest and the intestinal fraction moves the slowest.

Q5. Which isoenzyme is the most heat resistant and which one is the most heat labile?
Ans. Placental ALP is the most heat stable (resist heat at 65°C for 30 min) and bone ALP is the most heat labile.

Q6. What is Regan isoenzyme?
Ans. Regan isoenzyme is special isoenzyme which is seen in 3 to 15% of cancer patients and is referred as carcinoplacental alkaline phosphatase.

For more questions and answers of LFT, please refer Chapter 11.

Notes

CHAPTER

16

Estimation of Total Protein in Serum and Other Biological Fluids

> **Competency**
>
> **BI 11.8, 11.21:** Demonstrate estimation of serum proteins.

There are many proteins in the plasma. They play diverse role, e.g. they transport protein, help in clotting process, and play role in immunity.

Under the heading of total protein assessment, all these diverse proteins circulating in the plasma are collectively measured.

Biuret Method

It is the most commonly used method for estimation of total protein in clinical lab. Minimum of two peptide bonds are required for giving violet color chelate in presence of cupric ion, hence amino acid and dipeptide (Dipeptides are made up of two amino acids and have only one peptide bond.) do not react with cupric ion to give violet color chelate.

This method is called biuret method because a compound known as biuret ($NH_2CONHCONH_2$) reacts with cupric ion in similar manner to give colored complex.

Principle

Cupric ion (Cu^{++}) of $CuSO_4$ which is present in biuret reagent interacts with groups involved in making the peptide bond (NH-CO group) under alkaline medium. This results in formation of violet-colored complex, if minimum two peptide bonds are present. The absorbance of color developed is measured at 540 nm.

Color developed ranges between pink to various shades of purple depending upon the number of copper coordinate complex formed which in turn depends upon the number of peptide bond present in protein (size of protein).

Sodium potassium tartrate prevents precipitation of copper in alkaline medium and potassium iodide acts as an antioxidant.

Reagents Required

1. Biuret reagent [contain $CuSO_4$, NaOH, sodium potassium tartrate and potassium iodide)
2. Protein standard (280 mg/dL or 2.8 mg/mL)

Assay Procedure

Three test tubes are taken and marked as T, S, B. Reagents are added in these test tubes as per plan in Table 16.1.

Table 16.1: Scheme for estimation total protein by biuret method			
Reagents	B (blank) mL	S (standard) mL	T (test) mL
Serum			100 µL
Standard (280 mg/dL)		2.5	
DW	2.5		2.4
Biuret reagent	3.5	3.5	3.5
Total	6	6	6

Mix well and incubate at 37°C for 10 min (Fig. 16.1).
Read absorbance at 540 nm.

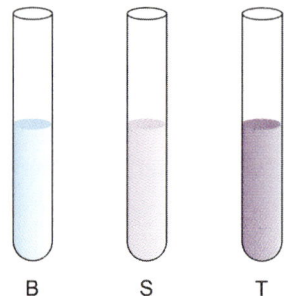

Fig. 16.1: Estimation of total protein by biuret method

Calculation

Concentration of protein in serum = OD of test/OD of standard × amount of standard (in mg)/volume of serum (in mL) × 100

OD of test/OD of standard × 7/0.1 × 100

[Amount of standard = 1 mL has 2.8 mg so 2.5 mL will have 2.8 × 2.5 = 7 mg]

OD of test/OD of standard × 7000 mg/dL

OD of test/OD of standard × 7 g/dL

Interpretation

Normal range:
- In male: 6.5 to 8.0 g/dL
- In female: 5.5 to 7.5 g/dL

[**Note:** Learner needs to pay attention that the unit of plasma protein is in gram per dL, unlike many other parameters like glucose, urea, creatinine, uric acid, bilirubin, cholesterol, etc. which are represented in mg per dL.]

Hypoproteinemia: Seen in following conditions:
- Liver disease: Due to lack of synthesis.
- Proteinuria: Loss in nephropathy, nephrotic syndrome

- Malnutrition: Poor intake of protein, so essential amino acids are deficient hence protein synthesis does not take place.
- Malabsorption
- Loss via skin (burn cases)

Hyperproteinemia: Seen in following conditions:
- Dehydration due to vomiting, diarrhoea, excess sweating
- Excess albumin infusion
- Multiple myeloma

Other methods of protein assessment are:
1. Kjeldahl method
2. Lowry method (Folin-Ciocalteu method/phosphotungstic-phosphomolybdic acid)
3. Direct photometric method: Absorption at 280 nm is assessed.
4. Dye binding method: Amido black 10 B dye or CBB
5. Refractometry
6. Turbidimetric method
7. Nephelometric method.

Estimation of Total Protein

Method Used: _____
_____
_____
_____

Observation

OD of blank: Adjusted to zero

OD of test: _____

OD of standard: _____

Calculation

Concentration of protein in serum = OD of test/OD of standard × Amount of standard (mg)/Volume of serum (mL) × 100 mg/dL

[Amount of standard = 1 mL has 2.8 mg so 2.5 mL will have 2.8 × 2.5 = 7 mg]

OD of test/OD of standard × 7/0.1 × 100 mg/dL

OD of test/OD of standard × 7000 mg/dL

OD of test/OD of standard × 7 g/dL

Result

_____
_____
_____

Clinical Correlation: _____
_____
_____
_____

Dated: _____   **Teacher's Signature**

VIVA VOCE

Q1. What all proteins constitute total protein?
Ans. Total protein consists of following proteins:
- Albumin
- Globulin
- Fibrinogen
- Transferrin
- Ceruloplasmin
- Alpha 1 antitrypsin
- Various clotting factors

Q2. What is the normal level of total protein in the serum in healthy adult?
Ans. Normal range of protein in plasma/serum:
- In male: 6.5 to 8.0 g/dL
- In female: 5.5 to 7.5 g/dL

Q3. What method may be used to separate different proteins in the plasma?
Ans. Electrophoresis

CHAPTER

17

Estimation of Albumin in Serum and Calculation of A:G Ratio

Competency

BI 11.8, 11.22: Demonstration of albumin estimation and calculation of A:G ratio.

- Albumin is the protein which is synthesized in the liver.
- It is the major protein in the plasma and is present in the highest concentration.
- Albumin has major contribution (to the extent of 80%) in deciding the intravascular fluid colloid osmotic pressure.
- Albumin binds with thyroid hormone, fatty acid, bilirubin, salicylates and many other drugs and help in their transportation in the plasma. Albumin is negative acute phase reactant protein.
- Following methods may be used for estimation of albumin:
  1. BCG (bromocresol green) method
  2. BCP (bromocresol purple) method

BCG (Bromocresol Green) Method

Principle

Albumin has pI 4.7; at pH below this, albumin is cation. BCG dye is an anionic dye which specifically binds with albumin at acidic pH and gives colored complex (yellow green to green blue). This color is read at 620 nm.

Reagents Required

1. BCG dye solution in succinate buffer
2. Normal saline
3. Standard of albumin (0.5 g/dL)

Assay Procedure

Three test tubes are taken and marked as B, S, T. Reagents are added in these test tubes as per plan in Table 17.1.

Mix tube well and keep at room temperature for 10 min.

[Dilute the serum in following manner: 1.8 mL of normal saline + 0.2 mL (200 µL) of serum = total volume 2 mL.]

Read at 620 nm.

Table 17.1: Scheme for estimation of albumin by BCG (bromocresol green) method			
Reagents	B (blank) mL	S (standard) mL	T (test) mL
Normal saline	0.2 mL		
Standard albumin (5 mg/mL)		0.2 mL	
Serum (diluted)			0.2 mL
BCG dye	5	5	5
Total	**5.2**	**5.2**	**5.2**

Calculation

Concentration of protein in serum = OD of test/OD of standard × Amount of standard (in mg)/Volume of serum (in mL) × 100

OD of test/OD of standard × 1/0.02 × 100

OD of test/OD of standard × 5000 mg/dL

OD of test/OD of standard × 5 g/dL

Interpretation

Normal range: Normal level of albumin in plasma is 3.5 to 5.5 g/dL.

Globulin calculation: Globulin can be assessed in plasma by using the formula given below.

Globulin = Total protein–Albumin

A:G Ratio (Albumin: Globulin Ratio)

- A:G ratio can be calculated as follow: Level of plasma albumin/level of plasma globulin
- Normal A:G ratio is 1.5: 1 to 2.5:1
- A:G ratio is reversed in:
  1. Multiple myeloma (due to excess globulin production)
  2. Chronic liver disease (low albumin production)
  3. Nephrotic syndrome (due to loss of albumin in the urine)

Estimation of Albumin

Method Used: _____

_____

_____

_____

Observation

OD of blank: Adjusted to zero

OD of test: _____

OD of standard: _____

Calculation

Concentration of albumin in serum = OD of test/OD of standard × Amount of standard (mg)/Volume of serum (mL) × 100 mg/dL

OD of test/OD of standard × 1/0.02 × 100 mg/dL

OD of test/OD of standard × 5000 mg/dL

OD of test/OD of standard × 5 g/dL

Result

_____

_____

_____

Clinical Correlation: _____

_____

_____

_____

Dated: _____   **Teacher's Signature**

VIVA VOCE

Q1. What is the normal level of albumin in healthy adult?
Ans. Normal level of albumin in plasma is 3.5 to 5.5 g/dL.

Q2. What is the role of albumin in the plasma?
Ans. Albumin has major contribution (to the extent of 80%) in deciding the intravascular fluid colloid osmotic pressure. Albumin binds with thyroid hormone, fatty acid, bilirubin, salicylates and many other drugs and helps in their transportation in the plasma. Albumin is negative acute phase reactant protein.

Q3. What is A:G ratio? What conditions A:G ratio is altered?
Ans.
- Ratio of plasma level of albumin and plasma level of globulin is known as A:G ratio.
- A:G ratio can be calculated as follow:
    – Level of plasma albumin/Level of plasma globulin
- Normal A:G ratio is 1.5: 1 to 2.5:1.
- A:G ratio is reversed in:
    1. Multiple myeloma (due to excess globulin production)
    2. Chronic liver disease (due to low albumin production)
    3. Nephrotic syndrome (due to loss of albumin in the urine)

Q4. Why albumin is predominantly lost in the urine in case of any nephropathy?
Ans. In normal health, negatively charged albumin is repelled by negatively charged basement membrane. Any disruption in intactness of basement membrane results in loss of negative charge on it and hence albumin is no more repulsed. In addition, learner should know that the size of albumin is smaller than globulin hence it is preferably filtered by glomerulus.

Q5. What is isoelectric pH (pI) and what is the value of pI of albumin?
Ans. pH at which protein has no net charge is known as isoelectric pH [pI]. pI of human albumin is 4.7.

Q6. How many types of globulin are found in the plasma? Give some examples of each.
Ans. There are four types of globulin in the plasma:
- **Alpha 1 globulin:** Alpha 1 antitrypsin, alpha 1 fetoprotein, alpha 1 glycoprotein
- Alpha 2 globulin: Ceruloplasmin, haptoglobin, alpha 2 macroglobulin
- Beta globulin: Transferrin, hemopexin, beta 2 microglobulin, C-reactive protein
- Gamma globulin: Immunoglobulin (IgG, IgA, IgM, IgD, IgE)

Q7. Mention any two methods by which proteins can be separated?
Ans. Proteins can be separated by electrophoresis and also by chromatography.

Notes

CHAPTER 18

Estimation of Total Cholesterol

Competency

BI 11.9: Demonstrate the estimation of serum total cholesterol.

CLINICAL OVERVIEW OF CHOLESTEROL

Cholesterol is 27-carbon tetracyclic structure having cyclopentanoperhydrophenanthrene ring (Fig. 18.1).

There are two types of cholesterol in the cell:
- Free cholesterol (physiologically active cholesterol constituting 30% of total cholesterol), and
- Esterified cholesterol (inert and storage form of cholesterol constituting 70% of total cholesterol).

Cholesterol in the body may be exogenous (dietary) or it may be endogenous (synthesized in tissues).

Assessment of cholesterol is important as hypercholesterolemia is associated with atherosclerotic disorder.

Methods Used

Following methods may be adopted to estimate total cholesterol in the plasma:
1. Chemical method (Zak's method)
2. Enzymatic method/cholesterol oxidase-peroxidase (CHOD-POD) method

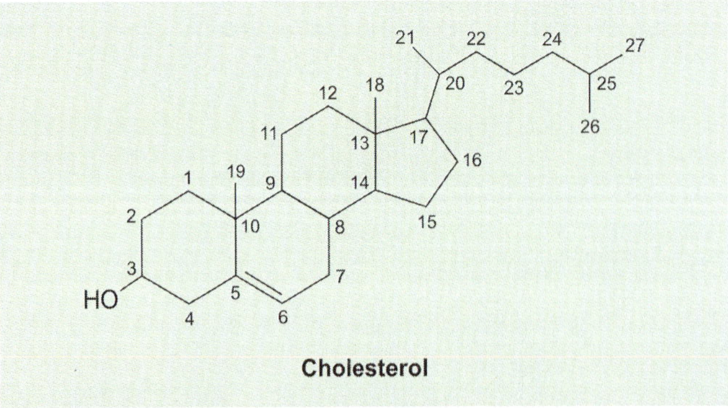

Fig. 18.1: Structure of cholesterol

Chemical Method (Zak's Method)

Principle

Cholesterol is acted upon by strong acid (concentrated H_2SO_4) and it undergoes **dehydration** followed by **oxidation and sulphonation** to produce reddish brown color complex. $FeCl_3$ acts as a catalyst in this reaction.

Red-colored complex is read at 540 nm.

Protein-free filtrate (PFF) is used for above reaction as protein tends to interfere with the reaction.

Reagents Required

1. Concentrated sulfuric acid
2. Acetic acid-ferric chloride reagent
3. Standard cholesterol: 200 mg/dL

Assay Procedure

Step 1: Preparation of PFF: Protein-free filtrate is prepared as per protocol given in Table 18.1.

Mix thoroughly with the stirrer for 15 min. Centrifuge at 3000 rpm for 3 min. Use supernatant for next step of actual color reaction.

Step 2: Actual color reaction: Three test tubes are taken and marked as B (blank), T (test), S (standard). Reagents are added in these tubes as per protocol given in Table 18.2.

- Mix well.
- Keep at water bath at 60°C for 10 minutes.
- Cool to room temperature.
- Read at 540 nm (Fig. 18.2)

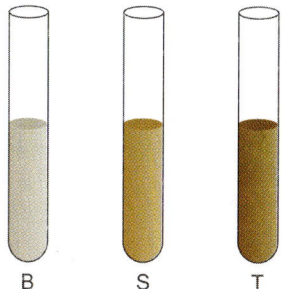

Fig. 18.2: Estimation of total cholesterol by Zak's method

Table 18.1: Preparation of PFF		
Reagent	T (mL)	S (mL)
$FeCl_3$—acetic acid reagent	9.8	9.8
Serum	0.2	
Standard cholesterol (200 mg/dL)		0.2
Total	**10**	**10**

Table 18.2: Scheme for estimation of total cholesterol by Zak's method			
Reagent	B (mL)	T (mL)	S (mL)
$FeCl_3$ reagent	5		
Test supernatant		5	
Standard supernatant			5
Conc H_2SO_4	3	3	3
Total	**8**	**8**	**8**

Calculation

Cholesterol concentration = OD of test/OD of standard × amount of standard*/volume of serum* × 100

OD of test/OD of standard × 0.2/0.1 × 100

OD of test/OD of standard × 2 × 100

OD of test/OD of standard × 200 mg%

*Amount of standard

- 10 mL of supernatant has 0.2 mL of standard, so 5 mL of supernatant has 0.1 mL of standard.
- 100 mL of standard has 200 mg of cholesterol, so 0.1 mL of standard will have 0.2 mg of cholesterol.

Volume of serum: 10 mL of supernatant has 0.2 mL of serum, so 5 mL of supernatant will have 0.1 mL of serum.

Enzymatic Method (Cholesterol Oxidase-Peroxidase Method/CHOD-POD Method)

- Cholesterol esterase first of all converts cholesterol ester to free cholesterol.
- Free cholesterol is then acted upon by cholesterol oxidase. H_2O_2 is the byproduct in this reaction catalysed by cholesterol oxidase.
- This H_2O_2 is then acted upon by peroxidase which produces nascent oxygen as a reactive species.
- Nascent oxygen then acts on 4 amino antipyrine to produce pink-colored complex 'quinoneimine' the concentration of which is read colorimetrically at 540 nm.

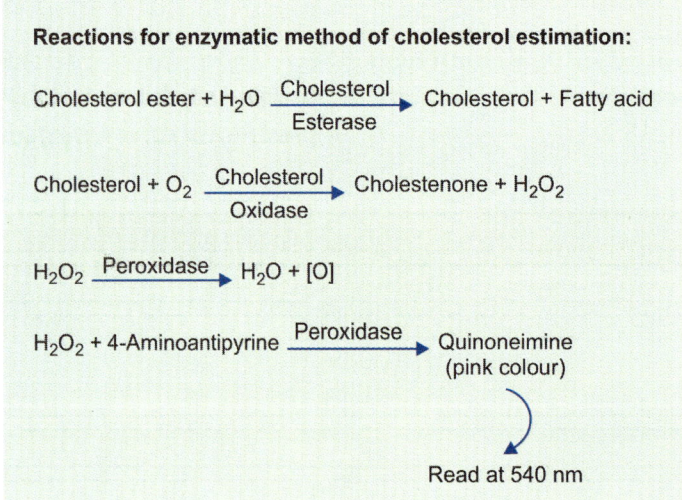

Fig. 18.3: Principle of cholesterol estimation

Interpretation

Desirable level of cholesterol in adults is <200 mg/dL.

Elevated in (hypercholesterolemia)

- Diabetes mellitus
- Nephrotic syndrome

- Type II hyperlipoproteinemia (familial hypercholesterolemia)
- Hypothyroidism
- Hypopituitarism

ASSESSMENT OF LDL

LDL cholesterol can be measured or can be calculated.

Measurement of LDL Cholesterol

Beta Quantification (Reference Method)
- Step 1: Ultracentrifugation to float VLDL and chylomicron.
- Step 2: Chemical precipitation of LDL from infranate obtained by ultracentrifugation.
- Step 3: Assessment of cholesterol in infranate from step 1. It gives the value of sum total of LDL and HDL cholesterol and assessment of cholesterol in supernatant from step 2 which gives the value of HDL cholesterol alone.
- Step 4: The LDL cholesterol is calculated by deducting the value of HDL cholesterol from sumtotal of LDL and HDL cholesterol.

Direct Method of Assessment of LDL

It uses immune separation, where latex beads coated with anti-VLDL and anti-HDL antibodies are used which bind with VLDL and HDL, respectively. This complex is then removed by centrifugation. The LDL cholesterol is then measured in remaining fluid by using appropriate method to estimate the cholesterol.

Calculation of LDL Cholesterol

Calculation of LDL Cholesterol Using Friedewald Formula

This formula gives accurate result of LDL cholesterol, if the level of TAG is less than 400 mg/dL.
1. HDL cholesterol is measured by direct or precipitation method.
2. Total cholesterol and TAG are measured.
3. VLDL is calculated as TAG/5.
4. Calculate/derive LDL(c) value using following formula:

$$LDL\ (C) = Total\ cholesterol - HDL\ (C) - TAG/5$$

Estimation of Cholesterol

Method Used: _____

_____

_____

_____

Observation

OD of blank: Adjusted to zero

OD of test: _____

OD of standard: _____

Calculation

Cholesterol concentration = OD of test/OD of standard × amount of standard/volume of serum × 100

OD of test/OD of standard × 0.2/0.1 × 100

OD of test/OD of standard × 2 × 100

OD of test/OD of standard × 200 mg%

Result

_____

_____

_____

Clinical Correlation: _____

_____

_____

_____

Dated: _____   **Teacher's Signature**

VIVA VOCE

Q1. What is the major contributor of total cholesterol in the plasma?
Ans. Total cholesterol is sum total of cholesterol present in various lipoproteins (LDL, HDL, VLDL).

Q2. What is the role of cholesterol in an extrahepatic cell?
Ans. In extrahepatic cell, cholesterol is important for making of cell membrane, steroid hormone synthesis.

Q3. What is the form of cholesterol which is transported by LDL in the plasma and which form it is delivered in the extrahepatic cell?
Ans. LDL transport cholesterol in cholesterol ester form in the plasma. But it delivers the cholesterol in extrahepatic cell in the form of free cholesterol.

Q4. What is the structure of cholesterol?
Ans. Cholesterol is 27-carbon compound which is made up of 4 rings known as cyclopentano-perhydrophenanthrene ring.

Cholesterol

Q5. What is the difference of cholesterol and cholesterol ester?
Ans. Cholesterol ester has fatty acid chain esterified at third hydroxyl group of cholesterol. Free cholesterol is amphipathic and cholesterol ester is a non-polar molecule.

Q6. How the dietary cholesterol is absorbed from intestinal lumen?
Ans. Dietary cholesterol (exogenous) is absorbed from intestinal lumen with the help of chylomicron.

Q7. Name the conditions where high level of cholesterol is found in the plasma.
Ans. Conditions where high cholesterol is found in plasma are:
- Diabetes mellitus
- Nephrotic syndrome
- Type II hyperlipoproteinemia (familial hypercholesterolemia)
- Hypothyroidism
- Hypopituitarism

Q8. What is the desirable level of various lipoproteins as per NCEP (ATP III) guidelines?
Ans.

ATP III classification of LDL, total, and HDL cholesterol (mg/dL)	
LDL cholesterol—primary target of therapy	
<100	Optimal
100–129	Near optimal/above optimal
130–159	Borderline high
160–189	High
≥190	Very high
Total cholesterol	
<200	Desirable
200–239	Borderline high
≥240	High
HDL cholesterol	
<40	Low
≥60	High

Q9. What all samples may be accepted for doing the lipid profile?
Ans. Following samples may be used for estimation of cholesterol:
a. Serum (red vacutainer)
b. EDTA plasma (purple vacutainer)

Q10. Name any other method which can be used to diagnose the type of dyslipoproteinemia in clinical labs.
Ans. Lipoprotein electrophoresis is an important technique which separates various lipoprotein in band fashion based on their charge and size. Agarose gel or polyacrylamide gel may be used for separation of lipoprotein. Densitometric assessment of these bands gives fair idea about the level of these lipoproteins in the plasma and helps in diagnosing the type of dyslipidemia patient may have.

Another method for separation and quantification of lipoprotein used in research laboratory is 'ultracentrifugation' which is based on density of lipoprotein. This is used in reference method for quantification of lipoproteins.

Notes

CHAPTER 19

Estimation of Triacylglycerol and HDL

> **Competencies**
>
> **BI 11.10:** Demonstrate the estimation of triglycerides (triacylglyceride).
> **BI 11.9:** Demonstrate the estimation of HDL-cholesterol.

CLINICAL OVERVIEW OF TRIACYLGLYCERIDE

Triacylglyceride in the body may be exogenous (dietary) or it may be endogenous (synthesized in tissues).

Method used for Assessment of Serum Triacylglyceride

Following enzymatic methods may be adopted to estimate triacylglyceride in the plasma.

Enzymatic Method

Following are the steps.
Step 1: Action of lipase

$$TAG + 3\ H_2O = glycerol + 3\ fatty\ acid$$

Step 2: Action of glycerol kinase

$$Glycerol + ATP = glycerolphosphate + ADP$$

Step 3: Action of glycerophosphate oxidase

$$Glycerolphosphate + O_2 = dihydroxyacetone + H_2O_2$$

Either H_2O_2 produced is measured by action of peroxidase enzyme which produces nascent oxygen (O) which acts on a dye (aminoantipyrine) to convert it to quinoneimine dye.

Or glycerophosphate can be measured by NADH production in a reaction, and this NADH is measured spectrophotometrically at 340 nm.

Interference

Endogenous plasma glycerol may give falsely high result of triacylglycerol. Glycerol may be high in plasma due to:
a. Infusion of IV fluids containing glycerol

b. Diabetes

c. Contamination of blood storage device

Reference method for TAG estimation: It involves alkaline hydrolysis, solvent extraction, and color reaction with chromotropic acid.

Interpretation

- Desirable level of triacylglyceride in adults is <200 mg/dL.
- Borderline high: 200 to 400 mg/dL.
- High: 400 to 1000 mg/dL
- Very high: >1000 mg/dL

Triacylglyceride elevated in (hypertriacylglyceridemia):

- Diabetes mellitus
- Nephrotic syndrome
- Type I hyperlipoproteinemia (familial hypertriacylglyceridemia)
- Type III, IV and type V hyperlipoproteinemias are also associated with elevated triacylglyceride level
- Hypothyroidism

ASSESSMENT OF HDL

Chemical Precipitation Method (Tedious and Outdated in Era of Automation)

A precipitation reagent (dextran sulfate + magnesium) is added to serum which precipitates and aggregates VLDL, LDL, CM (non-HDL lipoprotein). These non-HDL lipoproteins are then sedimented by centrifugation at the rate of 1500 rpm for 30 minutes. HDL cholesterol is then quantified in the supernatant by enzymatic method.

Homogenous Assay

In this technique, non-HDL lipoproteins are blocked by using certain polymers, detergents or modified enzyme in the first step and then HDL cholesterol is estimated using enzymatic method.

VIVA VOCE

Q1. What is the predominant source of TAG in the plasma?

Ans. Chylomicron is carrier of exogenous triacylglycerol in the plasma and VLDL is the carrier of endogenous triacylglycerol in the plasma.

Q2. What is the reason of lipemia in postprandial plasma?

Ans. The lipemia seen in postprandial plasma is due to chylomicron.

If the fasting sample is lipemic, it denotes abnormality and hints towards excess level of triacylglycerol in the plasma.

Q3. How the dietary triacylglycerol is absorbed from intestinal lumen?

Ans. Exogenous triacylglycerols are absorbed via chylomicrons which are organized in the intestinal mucosa.

Q4. What is ATP III classification of serum triacylglyceride (mg/dL)?

Ans.

ATP III classification of serum triacylglyceride (mg/dL)	
<150	Normal
150–199	Borderline high
200–499	High
≥500	Very high

Q5. Why HDL is known as good cholesterol?

Ans. HDL being called good cholesterol is actually a misnomer because HDL is a lipoprotein and not the cholesterol per se. It is said to be good because HDL is responsible for reverse cholesterol transport, thus removing the surplus cholesterol from extrahepatic tissues and protecting them.

Notes

CHAPTER

20

Estimation of Calcium

Competency

BI 11.11: Demonstrate estimation of calcium.

INTRODUCTION

Total content of calcium in a healthy adult is 1 to 1.5 kg. Approximately 99% of this calcium is in bone and teeth and rest is in other tissues and plasma.

Plasma calcium is in three forms:
1. Free or ionized form (50% of total plasma calcium)
2. Bound to protein (mainly albumin and also globulin) form (40% of total plasma calcium)
3. Bound to other anions like citrate, bicarbonate, lactate, phosphate and oxalate form (50% of total plasma calcium)

Ionized form of calcium is the active physiological form. Proteins are negatively charged at physiological plasma pH (7.35 to 7.45) and hence it binds calcium (Ca^{++}) avidly. Change in plasma pH alters the charge on protein and hence the binding of calcium to it.

For example, in alkalosis when plasma pH is increased, protein gets more of the negative charge enhancing the binding of calcium to it and reducing the free or ionized form of calcium. This results in hypocalcemia features.

Concentration of plasma protein also plays important role in distribution of calcium in free and bound forms. For example, in hypoalbuminemia, more of the calcium is in free or ionized form.

ROLE OF CALCIUM

Calcium plays important role in maintaining health. Important role of calcium is mentioned below.
- Contraction of muscle
- Acts as second messenger
- Needed for secretion of hormones
- Calcium is an important metallic cofactor which is required for action of many enzymes.
- Blood coagulation
- Bone and teeth formation

Estimation of Calcium

Level of Calcium in Serum in Health (Table 20.1)

Table 20.1: Total and ionized calcium in normal adult and normal child				
Age group	Total calcium		Ionized calcium	
	mg/dL	mmol/L	mg/dL	mmol/L
Adult	8.6 to 10	2.15 to 2.50	4.6 to 5.3	1.16 to 1.32
Child	8.8 to 10.8	2.20 to 2.70	4.8 to 5.5	1.20 to 1.38

Following are the important methods by which serum calcium can be measured.
 a. OCPC (O-cresolphthalein complexone) method (colorimetric method)
 b. Calcium-Arsenazo III dye method
 c. Method of Clark and Collip (titration method using $KMnO_4$)
Above methods estimate total calcium. Ionized calcium is measured by ISE (ion selective electrode).

Sample to be used:
- Serum or lithium heparin plasma is preferred sample for calcium estimation.
- EDTA and oxalate bind calcium ion, hence, cannot be used for assessment of calcium.

OCPC (O-Cresolphthalein Complexone) Method (Colorimetric Method)

Principle

In this method, a dye named O-cresolphthalein complexone is used which binds the calcium in alkaline medium to give pink-colored complex. The intensity of color which develops is measured at 580 nm (Fig. 20.1).

Analysis

Reagents required:
a. Coloring reagent: pH is alkaline (11.7)
 [O-cresolphthalein complexone + urea + ethanol + hydroxyquinoline + acetic acid in diethanolamine buffer]
b. Calcium standard: 10 mg/dL

Assay Procedure

- Three test tubes marked as T, B, S for test, blank and standard are taken and processed as given in Table 20.2.
- Test tubes are mixed well.
- Incubation at room temperature for 5 minutes.
- Absorbance is read at 580 nm.

Table 20.2: Scheme for estimation of calcium by OCPC method			
Reagents	Blank (mL)	Standard (mL)	Test (mL)
Coloring reagent	5	5	5
Standard (10 mg/dL)		0.5	
Serum (1:10 dilution)			0.5
DW	0.5		
Total	**5.5**	**5.5**	**5.5**

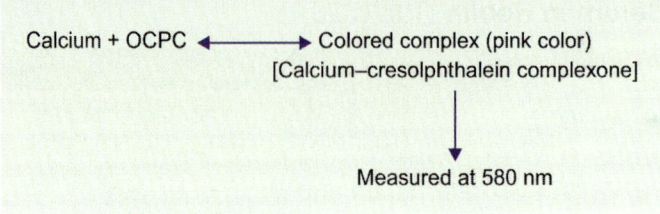

Fig. 20.1: Principle of calcium estimation

Calculation

Following formula applied for calculation:

Concentration of calcium in serum = OD of test/OD of standard × amount of standard (in mg)/volume of serum (in mL) × 100

Above method estimates amount of total calcium in the plasma.

OCPC method is commonly used method in clinical labs.

Calcium-Arsenazo III Dye Method

This is also commonly used in routine clinical lab. Here also colored complex is produced which is measured colorimetrically.

Method of Clark and Collip (Titration Method Using KMnO$_4$)

Principle

In this method, calcium is precipitated as calcium oxalate which is then titrated with potassium permanganate solution (KMnO$_4$). Precipitation of calcium as calcium oxalate is done with the help of ammonium oxalate. Before titration, calcium oxalate is dissolved in 1 N sulfuric acid to produce oxalic acid.

The end point of titration is indicated by development of pink color. The titer value is used to calculate the concentration of calcium.

It is a crude method of estimation of calcium and is not being used in clinical labs.

Estimation of Calcium

Method Used: _____
_____
_____
_____

Observation

OD of blank: Adjusted to zero

OD of test: _____

OD of standard: _____

Calculation

Concentration of calcium in serum = OD of test/OD of standard × amount of standard (in mg)/volume of serum (in mL) × 100

Result

_____
_____
_____

Clinical Correlation: _____
_____
_____
_____

Dated: _____   **Teacher's Signature**

VIVA VOCE

Q1. What is corrected calcium?
Ans. Plasma protein (specially albumin) has profound effect in determining the percentage of calcium which is in free (physiological) form and the one which is in bound form. Hence, the correction for plasma albumin is taken into consideration and corrected total calcium level is calculated. [Corrected total calcium is the value where the correction for protein variation is being done.]
Formula is:

Corrected total calcium (mg/dL) = total calcium + 0.8 (4-albumin in g%)

Q2. What is the normal value of total calcium and ionized calcium in a healthy adult.
Ans. Normal value of total and ionized calcium in adult and child

Age group	Total calcium		Ionized calcium	
	mg/dL	mmol/L	mg/dL	mmol/L
Adult	8.6 to 10	2.15 to 2.50	4.6 to 5.3	1.16 to 1.32
Child	8.8 to 10.8	2.20 to 2.70	4.8 to 5.5	1.20 to 1.38

Q3. Mention few common causes of hypocalcemia.
Ans. They are:
- Vitamin D deficiency
- Hypoparathyroidism
- Malabsorption
- Chronic renal failure

Q4. Mention few common causes of hypercalcemia.
Ans. They are:
- Hypervitaminosis D
- Hyperparathyroidism
- Multiple myeloma
- Milk alkali syndrome

Q5. Explain the effect of pH on level of ionized calcium in the plasma.
Ans. Ionized form of calcium is the active physiological form. Proteins are negatively charged at physiological plasma pH (7.35 to 7.45) and hence it binds calcium (Ca^{++}) avidly. Change in plasma pH alters the charge on protein and hence the binding of calcium to it. For example, in alkalosis when plasma pH is increased, protein gets more of the negative charge enhancing the binding of calcium to it and reducing the free or ionized form of calcium. Reverse is true in case of acidosis.

Q6. Name two commonly used methods to estimate total calcium in serum.
Ans. They are:
- Calcium-Arsenazo III dye method
- OCPC (O-cresolphthalein complexone) method

Above methods are colorimetric methods.

Q7. How the ionized calcium is measured?
Ans. Ionized calcium is measured using ion selective electrode (ISE).

Q8. What is the preferred sample for calcium estimation and why?
Ans. Sample to be used:
- Serum or lithium heparin plasma is preferred sample for calcium estimation.
- EDTA and oxalate bind calcium ion, hence cannot be used for assessment of calcium.

Notes

CHAPTER

21

Estimation of Phosphorus

Competency

BI 11.11: Demonstrate estimation of phosphorus.

INTRODUCTION

Phosphorus is found in organic and inorganic forms. Total content in healthy adult is 500 grams. Majority of it is in bone (90%).

Role of Phosphorus

1. Bone formation
2. Component of phospholipid, nucleic acid
3. Required in inorganic form in various metabolic pathways (glycolysis, glycogenolysis)
4. Needed for nucleotide formation (ATP, GTP, UDP, CTP, etc.)
5. Needed as a component of coenzyme (TPP, PLP)

Normal Range

- Adult: 2.5 to 4.5 mg/dL
- Children: 4 to 6 mg/dL

Sample to be Used

- Serum or lithium heparin plasma is preferred sample for phosphorus estimation.
- EDTA, citrate and oxalate cannot be used for assessment of phosphorus as they interfere with the assessment.
- Hemolyzed sample cannot be used as RBC contains high amount of phosphorus.
  Serum phosphorus can be measured by Fisk and Subba Rao Method.

Fisk and Subba Rao Method

Reagents Required

a. Acid molybdate reagent
b. H_2SO_4: 10 N
c. Trichloroacetic acid (10% W/V)

Estimation of Phosphorus

d. Reducing agent (amino naphthol sulfonic acid)
e. Phosphate standard: 0.8 mg/dL

Principle

PFF (protein-free filtrate) is prepared and is reacted with acid molybdate reagent to produce phosphomolybdic acid which is reduced to molybdenum blue. This blue color complex is read at 680 nm (red filter).

Assay Procedure

Preparation of PFF: 2 mL of serum and 8 mL of 10% TCA mixed in a tube which is then centrifuged. Supernatant is used as PFF.

Three test tubes marked as T, B, S for test, blank and standard are taken and processed as given in Table 21.1.

Table 21.1: Scheme of phosphorus estimation by Fisk and Subba Rao method

Reagents	Blank (mL)	Standard (mL)	Test (mL)
PFF			5
Standard (0.8/dL)		5	
Molybdate reagent	1	1	1
DW	5		
Reducing agent	0.4	0.4	0.4
Total	6.4	6.4	6.4

Test tubes are mixed well.
Incubation at room temperature for 5 minutes.
Absorbance is read at 680 nm.

Calculation

Following formula applied for calculation:

Concentration of phosphorus in serum = OD of test/OD of standard × amount of standard (in mg)/volume of serum (in mL) × 100

Estimation of Serum Phosphorus

Method Used: _____
_____
_____
_____

Observation

OD of blank: Adjusted to zero

OD of test: _____

OD of standard: _____

Calculation

Concentration of phosphorus in serum = OD of test/OD of standard × amount of standard (in mg)/volume of serum (in mL) × 100

Result

_____
_____
_____

Clinical Correlation: _____
_____
_____
_____

Dated: _____   **Teacher's Signature**

VIVA VOCE

Q1. What is the normal level of phosphorus?
Ans. Normal range:
- Adult: 2.5 to 4.5 mg/dL
- Children: 4 to 6 mg/dL

Q2. What sample can be used?
Ans. Sample to be used:
- Serum or lithium heparin plasma is preferred sample for phosphorus estimation.
- EDTA, citrate and oxalate cannot be used for assessment of phosphorus as they interfere with the assessment.
- Hemolyzed sample cannot be used as RBC contains high amount of phosphorus.

Q3. Common causes of hypophosphatemia.
Ans. They are:
- Hyperparathyroidism
- Fanconi syndrome
- Malabsorption
- Parenteral nutrition

Q4. Common causes of hyperphosphatemia.
Ans. They are:
- Hypoparathyroidism
- Renal failure
- Chemotherapy
- Rhabdomyolysis

Q5. What is the role of phosphorus in the body?
Ans. Role of phosphorus:
1. Bone formation
2. Component of phospholipid, nucleic acid
3. Required in inorganic form in various metabolic pathways (glycolysis, glycogenolysis)
4. Needed for nucleotide formation (ATP, GTP, UDP, CTP, etc.)
5. Needed as a component of coenzyme (TPP, PLP)

Notes

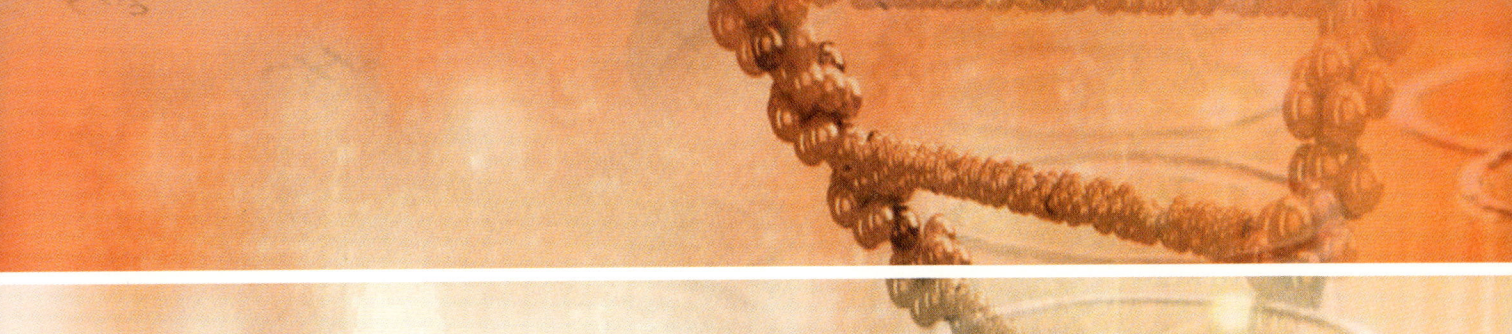

Section IV

Organ Function Tests

22. Thyroid, Pancreatic and Gastric Function Tests

CHAPTER 22

Thyroid, Pancreatic and Gastric Function Tests

Competencies

BI 6.14: Describe the tests that are commonly done in clinical practice to assess the functions of thyroid gland.
PY 4.8: Describe and discuss gastric function tests, pancreatic exocrine function tests.

Following function tests will be described in this chapter:
1. Thyroid function test
2. Pancreatic function test
3. Gastric function test

THYROID FUNCTION TEST

Thyroid gland is responsible for secretion of thyroid hormone and calcitonin. Thyroid hormone is needed for regulating various metabolism, neurological development and other functions in body and calcitonin is important for regulation of calcium metabolism.

Thyroglobulin is a glycoprotein found in colloid of thyroid follicle. Thyroglobulin is rich in tyrosine amino acid.

Iodine Uptake and Thyroid Hormone Synthesis by Thyroid Follicular Cell

It is described in Figure 22.1.

Majority of secreted T_4 (80%) is metabolized to T_3 and rT_3. Figure 22.2 is denoting how this conversion takes place.

In circulation, majority of T_4 and T_3 are bound to binding protein and are unavailable for metabolic role. It is only the free fraction of these hormones (FT_4 and FT_3) which are available for metabolic role.

In a normal healthy non-pregnant adult, only 0.04% of T_4 and 0.4% of T_3 are in free (unbound) form and are metabolically available for action.

Thyroid hormone binding proteins are:
1. Thyroxine binding globulin (TBG)
2. Thyroxine binding prealbumin (TBPA)
3. Albumin

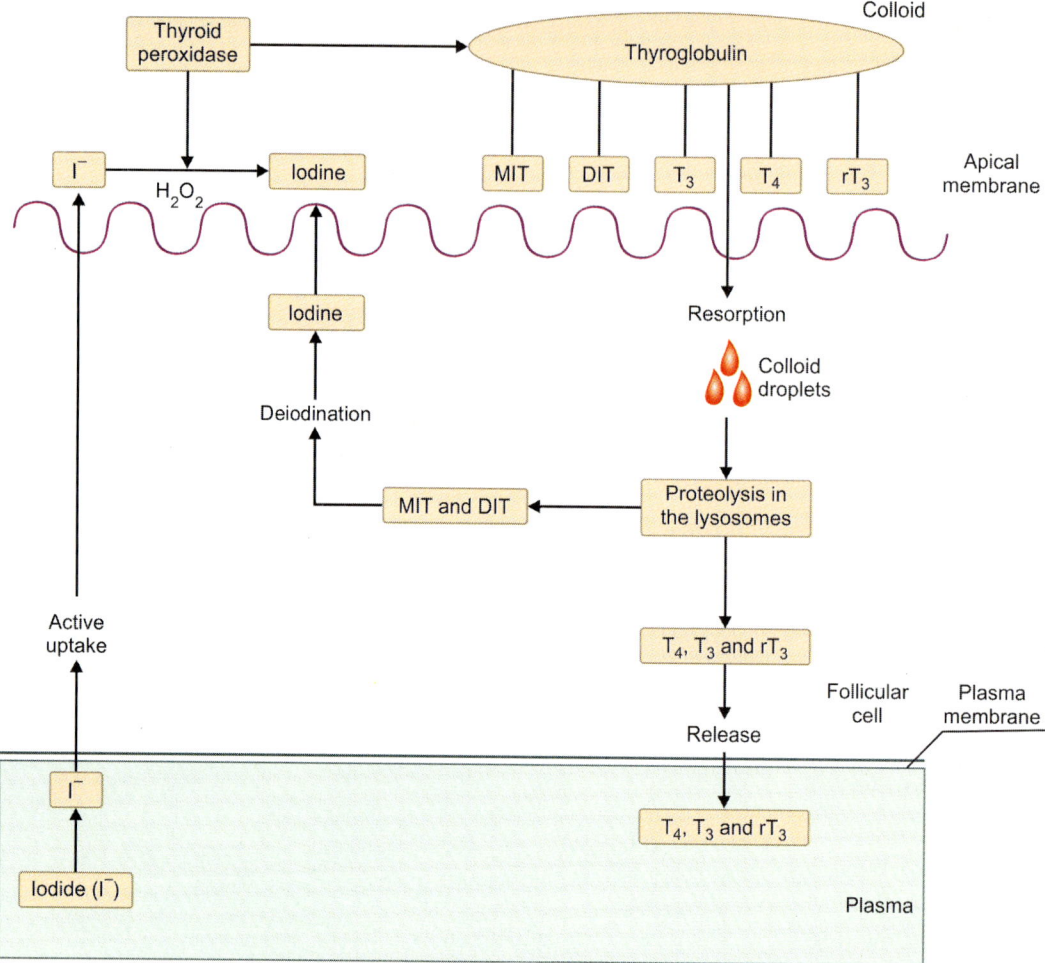

Fig. 22.1: Formation of thyroid hormone (T_4 and T_3) by thyroid follicular cell

Control of Thyroid Hormone Secretion

Hypothalamic-pituitary-thyroid axis is important in regulation of thyroid hormone secretion (Fig. 22.3).

Thyroid Function Tests

To evaluate the functioning of thyroid gland, following blood tests are being done:
1. TSH
2. FT_3
3. FT_4

TSH: Most sensitive method of detection of TSH is chemiluminometric immunoassay (CLIA) where detection limit is 0.01 mIU/L and so it is less likely to give false negative result.

FT_3 and FT_4: Free fractions of T_3 and T_4 (unbound form) (FT_3 and FT_4) are biologically active and are preferentially being estimated for assessing thyroid function over the total T_3 and total T_4. Values of total T_3 and T_4 change depending upon level of binding proteins, (irrespective of thyroid disease) hence are not being preferred to assess thyroid function.

Again, CLIA is preferred method of FT_3 and FT_4 estimation.

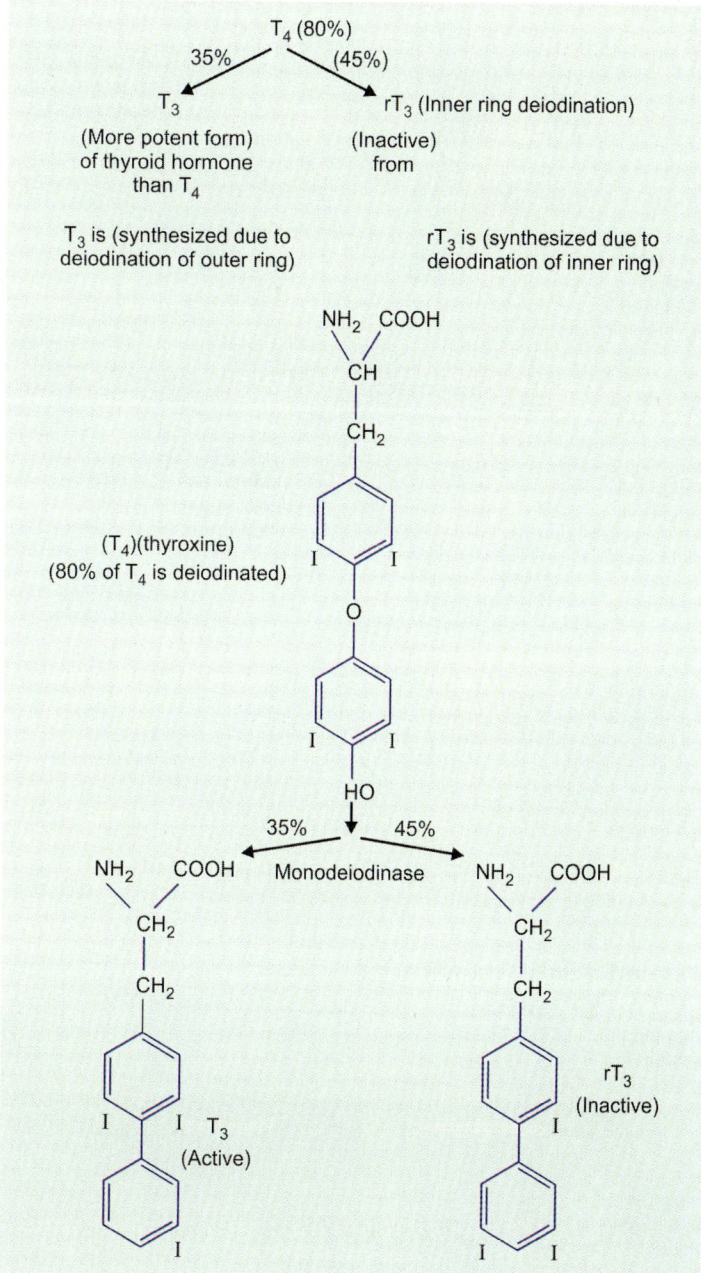

Fig. 22.2: Deiodination and conversion of T_4 to T_3 and rT_3

Hypothyroidism

Hypothyroidism is defined as low level of FT_4 with simultaneous high or normal level of TSH. Hypothyroidism is most common thyroid disorder affecting >5% of adult population.

Women are more prone to develop hypothyroid and risk increases with age. Important clinical symptoms of hypothyroidism are cold intolerance, weight gain, constipation, dry skin, menorrhagia. Signs are bradycardia, diastolic hypertension, periorbital edema, delayed deep tendon reflex.

Hypothyroidism can be classified as primary, secondary and tertiary based on location of defect which results in hypothyroidism **(Fig. 22.4)**.

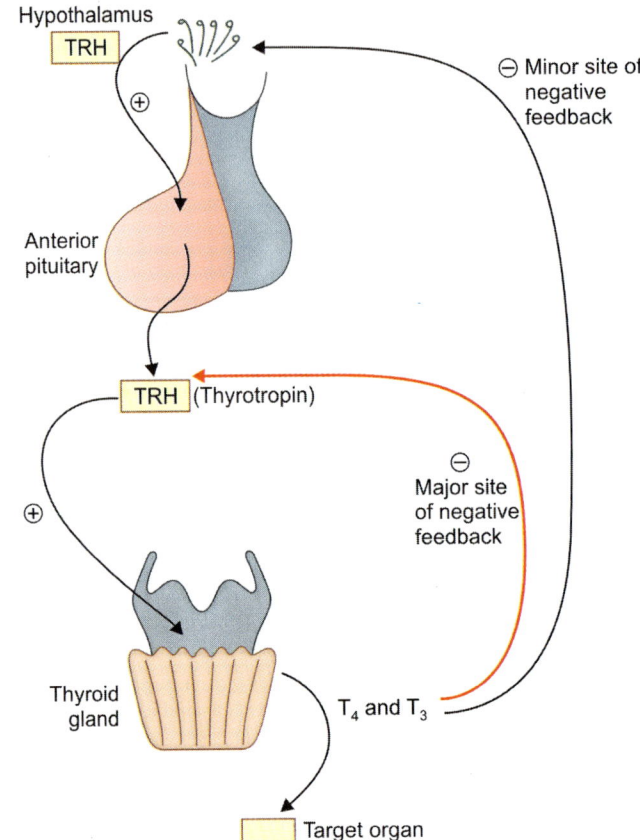

Fig. 22.3: Hypothalamic-pituitary-thyroid axis

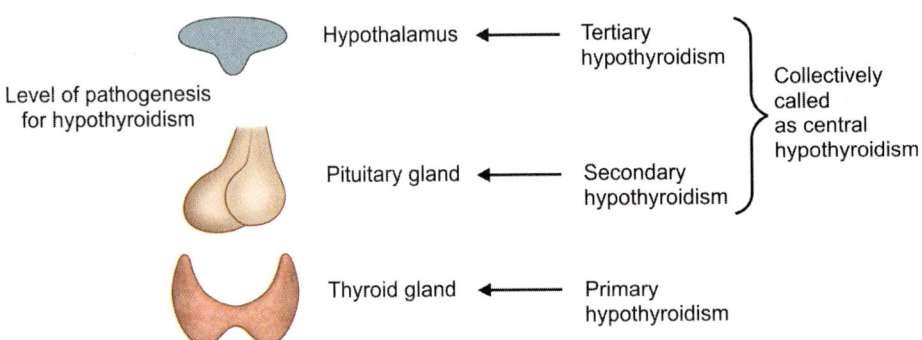

Fig. 22.4: Level of involvement in primary, secondary and tertiary hypothyroidism

Primary: Here the defect lies at the level of thyroid gland which is not able to produce thyroid hormone adequately.

Causes for **primary hypothyroidism** are enlisted below:
1. Iodine deficiency
2. Chronic autoimmune thyroiditis (atrophic and goitrous form)
3. Total or subtotal thyroidectomy
4. Infiltrative disorders (sarcoidosis, amyloidosis, lymphoma)

5. Thyroid dysgenesis
6. Congenital defect in thyroid hormone biosynthesis
7. Drugs: Lithium, radio tropic contrasts

On investigation, levels of FT_4 and FT_3 are found low, with the compensatory increase of TSH.

Central hypothyroidism: Here thyroid gland is otherwise normal, but it is not able to produce thyroid hormone (T_4 and T_3) adequately due to insufficient stimulation by TSH either due to disease of pituitary when TSH is not secreted adequately **(secondary hypothyroidism)** or else it may be due to inadequate production of thyrotropin release hormone (TRH) from hypothalamus which then is reflected in low TSH and **low FT_3 and FT_4 (tertiary hypothyroidism)**.

On investigation, in both secondary and tertiary hypothyroidisms, level of TSH and level of FT_4 and FT_3 are found low.

To differentiate secondary and tertiary hypothyroidism, TRH evaluation need to be done.
Normal values of TSH, FT_3 and FT_4:
- TSH = 0.35–5.0 mIU/L [µIU/mL]
- FT_4 = 0.50–1.40 ng/dL
- FT_3 = 1.8–4.20 pg/mL

Overt hypothyroidism *vs* subclinical hypothyroidism:
- *Overt hypothyroidism* [$\downarrow FT_4$ and TSH]: It is defined as low serum FT_4 and high serum TSH concentration.
- *Subclinical hypothyroidism*: It is defined as a normal serum FT_4 concentration and high (usually <10 mIU/mL) of TSH.

Treatment of Hypothyroidism

1. Treatment for the underlying cause whenever feasible
2. Supplementation of thyroxine [levothyroxine sodium]

Hyperthyroidism

Hyperthyroidism is less common compare to hypothyroidism.

Hyperthyroidism is defined as high serum level of FT_4 with simultaneous low or normal level of TSH. This is due to excessive synthesis of thyroid hormone from thyroid gland and its secretion.

Central Hyperthyroidism

Excess TSH is very rare cause of hyperthyroidism. Thyrotoxicosis is clinical manifestation of hyperthyroidism where there is a state of hypermetabolism. It is characterized by irritability, tremors, palpitations, weight loss, heat intolerance, etc. On examination, patient has tachycardia, tremors, ophthalmopathy (Graves' disease).

Causes of thyrotoxicosis:

1. Graves' disease [production of thyroid stimulator antibody (TSH R-stimulating antibody)]
2. Toxic nodular goitre
3. Toxic adenoma
4. TSH secreting tumor.

Treatment: Antithyroid drug (methimazole) is the mainstay of treatment.

PANCREATIC FUNCTION TEST

Exocrine function of pancreas is to secrete pancreatic fluid of pH 8.0 to 8.3 which consists of bicarbonate and enzymes like amylase, lipase, trypsin, etc.

24-hour volume of pancreatic juice may be as high as 3 liters. This pancreatic juice helps in considerable digestion and absorption of carbohydrate, lipid and protein. Disorders of exocrine pancreas are thus manifested as diarrhea and steatorrhea.

Pancreatic Disorders

Both in childhood and adult, there are many diseases which affect the functioning of exocrine pancreas.

1. Pancreatic disorders in childhood
- Morphogenesis disorder
  - Annular pancreas
  - Pancreas divisum
  - Pancreatic hypoplasia
  - Pancreatic agenesis
- Inherited syndrome: Cystic fibrosis
- Isolated enzyme deficiency.
- Acquired pancreatitis in childhood
  - Idiopathic
  - Traumatic
  - Drugs

2. Adult disorders of the exocrine pancreas causing pancreatitis
- Causes of acute pancreatitis in adult may be:
  - Gallstone
  - Alcohol
  - Infections (mumps, coxsackie B)
  - Pancreatic tumors
  - Drugs (azathioprine, estrogen, steroids)
  - Postsurgical
- Causes of chronic pancreatitis in adult may be:
  - Alcohol
  - Nutritional
  - Trauma
  - Idiopathic
  - Hypercalcemia

Test of Exocrine Pancreatic Function

Both invasive and non-invasive tests are being done to assess exocrine pancreatic function.

Non-invasive tests (tubeless) are easier to do but they lack sensitivity and specificity compared to invasive test.

Both are described below.

Invasive Test of Exocrine Pancreas

Total volume as well as the content of bicarbonate, amylase, lipase, trypsin is measured in duodenal fluid collected after giving **"Lundh Meal" which consists of 6% fat, 15% carbohydrate and 74% of non-nutrient fiber.**

This meal provides stimulus for pancreatic secretion but this test is of mere historical interest.

Secretin-cholecystokinin or secretin-ceruletide tests are considered as gold standard tests for assessing exocrine pancreatic function.

In this test, secretin injection is given IV followed by CCK (or ceruletide which is functional C-terminal cholecystokinin octapeptide sequence of intact hormone) injection and assessment of bicarbonate and enzymes in collected pancreatic juice is done.

Non-Invasive Test for Assessment of Exocrine Pancreatic Function

None of such non-invasive tests has adequate sensitivity. Due to large functional reserve of pancreas, there is considerable overlap of result of such tests with the normal person and those having pancreatic disease.

Pancreatic insufficiency cannot be demonstrated until at least 50% of the acinar cells are destroyed, and for being clinically symptomatic 90% of acinar cell must have destroyed.

Following tests are included under this heading:
1. **Fecal elastase test:** Reduction in level of fecal enzyme may be used as a marker of pancreatic insufficiency. It is the method of choice for non-invasive assessment of pancreatic insufficiency.
2. **^{13}C mixed chain triglyceride breath test:** Labelled ^{13}C fatty acid containing mixed triglyceride is given orally and breath is tested for labelled $^{13}CO_2$. If lipase enzyme is sufficient in intestinal lumen, then adequate amount of ^{13}C will be exhaled in breath. In case of pancreatic insufficiency, breath will have absence of ^{13}C labelled CO_2.

GASTRIC FUNCTION TEST

Main function of stomach is transient storage of food, churning and digestion. To find out gastric dysfunction, there are certain laboratory investigations which are carried out even today despite of advancement in endoscopic procedures which help direct visualization of interior of gastro-intestinal tract.

Tests for *Helicobacter pylori* (*H. pylori*) Infection

H. pylori is a spiral-shaped bacterium which tends to localize largely in gastric antrum. In 1985, association of *H. pylori* infection with peptic ulcer disease was described. Since then, a number of tests have been proposed to diagnose the infection by *H. pylori*. According to a report, 80% of Indian population seem to have infection by *H. pylori*; but only minority of such population develop peptic ulcer disease.

Major concern is that the *H. pylori* infection increases the risk of getting gastric malignancy manifold.

H. pylori produces **'urease' enzyme which breaks urea to bicarbonate and ammonia** which are important for survival of this organism in the stomach. This characteristic of *H. pylori* is the basis of **'urea breath test' and 'direct urease test'** on gastric biopsy specimen.

Urea Breath Test for H. pylori

This is the most widely used non-invasive test for detection of *H. pylori* infection.

Patient is given urea ^{13}C labelled as capsule or drink. If the patient is infected with *H. pylori*, this urea is converted to bicarbonate and ammonia. This bicarbonate has ^{13}C and is absorbed from stomach to blood and is broken down to $^{13}CO_2$ which is exhaled. Mass spectrometry detects $^{13}CO_2$ in breath sample collected 45 to 60 minutes after drinking the labelled urea.

In absence of *H. pylori* infection, when urease is absent in intestinal lumen, labelled urea is absorbed intact in the blood and is excreted as such in the urine.

Serological Test for H. pylori Infection

H. pylori specific antibodies (IgG and IgA) can be detected.

PCR

PCR for detection of nuclear sequence specific of *H. pylori* is also available; which detects it in feces and saliva.

Test for Gastric Acid Secretion and Gastrinomas

Before discovery of *H. pylori*, patients with gastric or duodenal ulcer were extensively tested for basal and maximal acid output (BAO and MAO) in gastric juice analysis.

Even for possible gastrinoma, BAO and MAO were being assessed. Nowadays, many non-invasive tests and state to art technologies like plasma gastrin measurement, endoscopy, CT scan, MRI, PET, etc. have replaced the need of acid output estimation for diagnosis of gastrinomas.

Gastrin is mainly secreted by 'G' cell of antral mucosa and to a lesser extent by 'G' cell of the proximal duodenum and 'Δ' cell of the pancreatic cell.

Gastrin once secreted into the blood, it stimulates secretion of gastric acid, intrinsic factor, pepsinogens and pancreatic bicarbonate and enzymes.

Gastric acid output: It is estimated using standard alkali (0.1 N NaOH)

Basal acid output (BAP) and maximum acid output (MAO): Normal BAO is 1–2.5 mmol of acid per hour and MAO is 20–40 mmol/hour.

Note: Zollinger-Ellison syndrome consists of
a. Multiple peptic ulcer
b. Gastric hypersecretion
c. Non-β islet cell tumors of the pancreas secreting gastrin.

Notes

Notes

Section V

Clinical Lab Patient's Report Interpretation (Chart Discussion/Spotter)

23. Enzyme as a Marker of Disease
24. Interpretation of Laboratory Result: Carbohydrate Metabolism
25. Interpretation of Laboratory Result: Oral Glucose Tolerance Test (OGTT)
26. Interpretation of Laboratory Result: Amino Acid Metabolism
27. Interpretation of Laboratory Result: Lipid Metabolism
28. Interpretation of Laboratory Result: Protein Metabolism
29. Interpretation of Laboratory Result: Purine Nucleotide Metabolism
30. Interpretation of Laboratory Result: Arterial Blood Gas (ABG) Analysis
31. Cerebrospinal Fluid (CSF)

CHAPTER 23

Enzyme as a Marker of Disease

Competency

BI 2.7: Interpret laboratory results of enzyme activities and describe the clinical utility of various enzymes as markers of pathological conditions.

Following case reports will be described under this heading:
- Myocardial infarction
- Acute pancreatitis
- Prostate cancer
- Prehepatic jaundice
- Hepatic jaundice
- Obstructive jaundice

Case: Myocardial Infarction

A 59-year-old male comes to emergency OPD with complain of severe pain towards left side of chest which is radiating to left arm and back for past 4 hours. He has the feeling of constriction in the chest. His father died at the age of 67 due to cardiac arrest.

Following were blood report of the patient:
- CPK (total): 210 U/L (N = 40–170 U/L)
- CPK (MB): 20 U/L (N = 3 to 10 U/L)
- CPK MB fraction was approximately 7.5% of total CPK compared to normal fraction of <5%.
- AST = 85 IU/L (normal = **0–35 IU/L**)
- Cardiac troponin I = Raised
- High-sensitive cardiac troponin T (hsTnT) = Raised

Comment on the clinical condition in this patient.

Explanation

This patient is suffering from myocardial infarction justified by typical clinical history and raised cardiac markers (TnT and TnI), CPK, etc.

Figure 23.1 and Table 23.1 explain the time of rise, peak and duration of enzyme elevation in a case of uncomplicated myocardial infarction (MI).

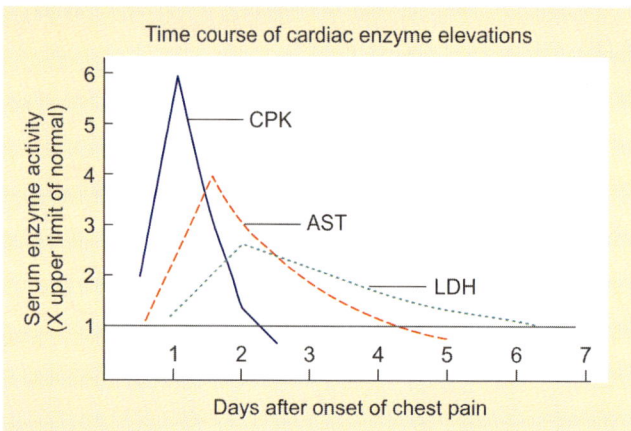

Fig. 23.1: Cardiac enzyme profile in serum after an episode of MI

Table 23.1: Cardiac enzymes: Time of rise, peak and duration in serum				
Marker	Normal value	Time when it starts increasing	Peak seen at	Persist till
CPK (CK)	40–170 U/L	3–6 hr	24–36 hr	3 to 4 days
AST	0–35 IU/L	8–12 hr	24 hr	3 to 6 days
LDH	55–140 IU/L	12–24 hr	48 to 72 hr	10 to 14 days
Troponins	Not detectable	3–12 hr	18-24 hr	10 days

Case: Acute Pancreatitis

A 65-year-old chronic alcoholic presents with excruciating pain in epigastric region of the abdomen which is radiating to back. Patient feels comfortable in sitting in squatting position. On examination, patient was in distress with low grade fever, bowel sounds were diminished and abdomen was distended.

Blood investigation showed:
- Serum amylase: 400 Somogyi units/100 mL (Normal: 80–180 Somogyi units/100 mL)
- Serum lipase: 110 U/L (Normal: 5–45 U/L)
- Random blood glucose: 198 mg/dL

Comment on the clinical condition in this patient.

Explanation

This patient may be suffering from acute pancreatitis. Most common cause of acute pancreatitis is gallbladder stone followed by chronic alcohol intake.

Diagnosis is established in presence of any two out of following three criteria:
1. Epigastric pain radiating to back
2. Threefold or greater elevation of serum lipase/amylase
3. Imaging abdomen shows acute pancreatitis.

Serum lipase is more specific for pancreatitis compared to serum amylase activity.

Case: Prostate Cancer

A 65-year-old male presents with complain of frequent urination and urinary incontinence. Digital rectal examination revealed firm and enlarged prostate.

Prostate specific antigen (PSA) assessment in blood gives the value of 50 ng/mL. (Normal is <4 ng/mL.)

Comment on the diagnosis.

Explanation

This patient has prostate gland enlargement which may be either due to BPH (benign prostatic hyperplasia) or may be because of prostate cancer. Both these conditions give elevated values of PSA.

Diagnosis is confirmed by prostate biopsy.

Case: Prehepatic (Hemolytic) Jaundice

A 10-year-old child is coming with history of extreme tiredness, lethargy, recurrent episodes of excruciating pain in lower limbs. History of passing normal-colored urine and dark-colored faeces is obtained. On examination, he is found to be anemic with yellowish discoloration of sclera and mucous membrane. Abdomen was tender with mild hepatomegaly.

The biochemical findings of the patient are as follows:

Serum	
Bilirubin (total)	10.0 mg/dL
Conjugated bilirubin	0.5 mg/dL
Unconjugated bilirubin	9.5 mg/dL
AST (SGOT)	28 IU/L (0–35 IU/L)
ALT (SGPT)	35 IU/L (0–35 IU/L)
ALP	45 IU/L ((30–120 IU/L)
Urine	
Bile pigments	Negative
Bile salts	Negative
Urobilinogen	+++
Stool	
Stercobilinogen	+++

1. Identify the most probable type of jaundice in this case, and justify your diagnosis.
2. Give one cause for this type of jaundice.

Explanation

1. This patient is most probably suffering with prehepatic (hemolytic) jaundice. Raised levels of unconjugated bilirubin in the plasma with normal level of conjugated bilirubin suggest that there is no obstruction in the excretion of conjugated bilirubin via bile, this rules out the obstructive jaundice.

    Liver enzymes are also within the normal limits which rules out hepatic cause of jaundice.

    Visible pallor and excruciating pain in the lower limbs are suggestive of sickle cell disease as a probable cause of hemolytic jaundice. This needs to be confirmed electrophoresis where HbS band is seen.
2. Sickle cell disease is an important cause of hemolytic jaundice. Deficiency of G6PD is also an important cause of hemolysis and prehepatic jaundice. In addition, malarial parasite causes considerable hemolysis and patient may present with features of prehepatic jaundice in malaria.

Case: Hepatic Jaundice

A 24-year-old male executive presents with fever, headache, nausea, loss of appetite and yellow discoloration of skin for past 2 days. History of passing yellow-colored urine and normal-colored faeces is obtained. On examination, mild hepatomegaly was found.

The biochemical findings of the patient are as follows:

Serum
Bilirubin (total)	7.0 mg/dL (0.3–1.0 mg/dL)
Conjugated bilirubin	2.5 mg/dL (0.1–0.3 mg/dL)
Unconjugated bilirubin	4.5 mg/dL (0.2–0.7 mg/dL)
SGOT (AST)	1200 IU/L (0–35 IU/L)
SGPT (ALT)	980 IU/L (0–35 IU/L)
Alkaline phosphatase	150 IU/L (30–120 IU/L)

Urine
Bilirubin	+
Bile salts	+
Urobilinogen	++

Stool
Stercobilinogen	++

1. **Identify the most probable type of jaundice in this case, and justify your diagnosis.**
2. **Enumerate two probable causes of the above biochemical picture.**

Explanation

Patient is suffering with hepatic jaundice. History of fever is suggestive of infective origin. Conjugation of bilirubin is affected in jaundice of hepatic origin due to lack of function of conjugating enzyme 'glucuronyl transferase'. Conjugated bilirubin is also considerably increased due to obstruction of bile flow because of edematous hepatocytes which block the liver sinusoids.

Raised transaminases (AST, ALT) support the diagnosis.

Common causes of hepatic jaundice are:
- Viral infection
- Drug toxicity
- Organic solvent toxicity

Case: Obstructive Jaundice

A 45-year-old lady is admitted with the complain of severe abdominal pain in upper right quadrant. History reveals that patient is passing high-colored urine and clay-color stool for past 5 days. Examination revealed yellow discoloration of sclera and skin. Scratch marks noticed all over the skin.

The biochemical findings of the patient are as follows:

Serum
Bilirubin (total)	10.0 mg/dL
Conjugated bilirubin	8.5 mg/dL
Unconjugated bilirubin	1.5 mg/dL
AST (SGOT)	28 IU/L (0–35 IU/L)
ALT (SGPT)	35 IU/L (0–35 IU/L)
ALP	340 IU/L (30–120 IU/L)

Urine	
Bile pigments	++
Bile salts	++
Urobilinogen	Negative
Stool	
Stercobilinogen	Negative

1. **Identify the most probable type of jaundice in this case, and justify your diagnosis.**
2. **Give at least two common causes of such type of jaundice.**
3. **What test is being done to find out the presence or absence of bilirubin, bile salt, urobilinogen in the urine?**

Explanation

1. This patient is suffering from 'obstructive jaundice'. It is said so because in obstructive jaundice conjugated bilirubin is increased in plasma due to obstruction in bile flow which results in regurgitation of conjugated bilirubin in the plasma. Conjugated bilirubin is water soluble; hence, it is excreted in urine giving dark color to the urine. Urobilinogen and stercobilinogen are not formed in the intestinal lumen due to lack of bilirubin in the intestinal lumen due to obstruction of bile flow; this results in lack of urobilinogen in the urine and clay-colored stool.

    Liver transaminases (AST and ALT) levels are normal as the hepatocytes are not damaged, but ALP is increased in obstructive jaundice.

2. Common causes of obstructive jaundice are stone in the biliary tract, stricture of duct, malignancy of head of pancreas.
3. Following tests are being done to find out above constituents in the urine:
   - Bilirubin: Fouchet's test
   - Bile salt: Hay's sulfur test
   - Urobilinogen: Ehrlich test

Notes

CHAPTER 24

Interpretation of Laboratory Result: Carbohydrate Metabolism

Competencies

BI 3.8: Discuss and interpret laboratory results of analytes associated with metabolism of carbohydrates.
BI 3.10: Interpret the results of blood glucose levels and other laboratory investigations related to disorders of carbohydrate metabolism.

Case: McArdle Disease

A 9-year-old boy presents to the OPD with exercise intolerance, easy tiredness and painful cramps for past one year. Following were the biochemical reports:
- Blood glucose: 100 mg/dL
- Blood lactate: 0.3 mmol/L (normal lactate: 0.5–1 mmol/L)
  Muscle biopsy showed excess glycogen (>4%).

1. **What is the probable diagnosis?**
2. **Biochemical basis of the sign and symptoms?**

Explanation

This boy is suffering from McArdle disease as specified by increased glycogen content in the muscle and low lactate level in the blood. In this disease, muscle glycogen phosphorylase is deficient resulting in the exercise intolerance as muscle glycogen is not able to provide required glucose-6-phosphate for glycolysis.

Blood lactate level is low after exercise due to obvious reason as there is no glycolysis is taking place in the muscle due to lack of glucose-6-phosphate.

Normal content of glycogen in the muscle is <1%, in McArdle disease the content of glycogen may go as high as >4%.

Second wind phenomenon is observed in McArdle disease, it is characterized by the patient's better tolerance for aerobic exercise such as walking and cycling after approximately 10 minutes of continued exercise. This is due to increased blood flow during early phase of exercise which provides fuel like glucose and fatty acid for sustaining the muscle exercise.

Case: Von Gierke Disease

A 10-year-old presents with enlarged abdomen, weakness, sweating and tremors. History of delayed developing milestones was found. On examination, liver was enlarged. On blood examination, following were reported:

- Fasting blood glucose: 49 mg/dL (severe hypoglycemia)
- Ketone bodies in urine: ++
- Blood lactate: 4.6 mmol/L (normal lactate-0.5–1 mmol/L)
- pH: 7.30
- Uric acid: 9.1 mg/dL

1. What is the probable diagnosis and biochemical?
2. What is the enzyme defect and biochemical basis of the sign and symptoms?

Explanation

This baby is suffering with **Von Gierke disease** which is **glycogen storage disorder Ia**. In this disease, there is deficiency of glucose-6-phosphatase which is the terminal enzyme of not only liver glycogenolysis but also of gluconeogenesis. This results in severe hypoglycemia in the baby.

Severe hypoglycemia results in mobilization of free fatty acid from adipose cell triacylglycerol due to action of **'hormone sensitive lipase'** enzyme. Excessive fatty acid beta oxidation in liver results in ketone body production.

Accumulated glucose-6-phosphate in liver enters in glycolysis and increased flux of glucose-6-phosphate in glycolysis in constant oxygen supply results in anaerobic glycolysis (Crabtree effect) and lactic acidosis.

Uric acid is high because of overproduction and underexcretion.

Case: Cori Disease

A 3-year-old child brought by mother with complain of early morning hypoglycemia. On examination, liver was enlarged. Following were biochemical findings:
- Blood glucose: 56 mg/dL
- KFT and LFT normal.

Muscle biopsy showed glycogen polymer with little branching (limit dextrin).

Comment on possible glycogen storage disorder.

Explanation

This child may be having Cori's disease (limit dextrinosis) which is due to lack of 'debranching' enzyme in liver and muscle both (IIIa) or in liver (IIIb) alone.

This disease is characterized by delayed hypoglycemia and also exercise intolerance when muscle is also involved.

Case: Classical Galactosemia

A 3-month-old infant presents with history of poor feeding, vomiting, repeated attack of hypoglycemia. Body weight is low for age. Liver was enlarged and bilateral cataract was seen (Fig. 24.1).

Lab reports are as follow:
- Random blood sugar: 60 mg/dL
- Serum uric acid: 7.9 mg/dL
- Lactic acid: High

1. What is the probable diagnosis?
2. What is the enzyme defect?
3. Biochemical basis of the sign and symptoms?

Interpretation of Laboratory Result: Carbohydrate Metabolism

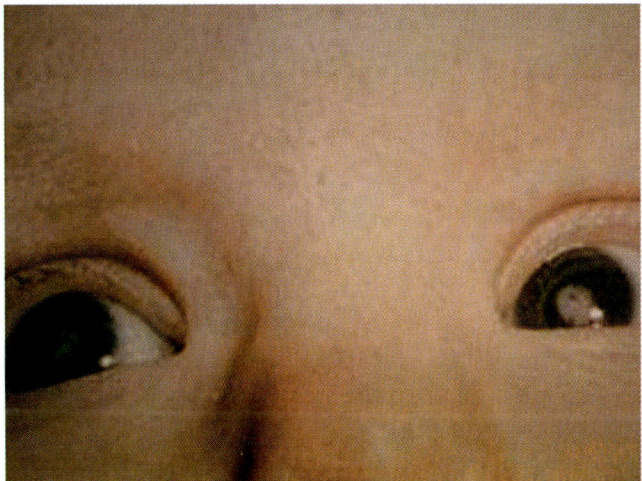

Fig. 24.1: Bilateral cataract in a case of classical galactosemia

Explanation

This baby is suffering with sign and symptoms suggestive of classical galactosemia, which is due to deficiency of **'galactose-1-phosphate uridyltransferase'** enzyme which is the exclusive enzyme of galactose metabolism.

Galactose-1-phosphate is accumulated in hepatocytes resulting in hepatomegaly and inhibition of glycogen phosphorylase enzyme by galactose-1-phosphate results in hypoglycemic attack.

Sequestration of ATP in conversion of galactose to galactose-1-phosphate results in increased purine nucleotide biosynthesis, degradation of which results in hyperuricemia. (ATP has inhibitory impact on purine nucleotide biosynthesis.)

Case: Diabetes Mellitus

A 47-year-old lady is coming with complain of increased thirst (polydipsia), increased appetite (polyphagia) and increased frequency of urine (polyuria) for past 6 months. Blood examination report is as follows:
- Fasting plasma glucose: 146 mg/dL
- Postprandial blood sugar: 209 mg/dL
- HbA1c: 7 %

Urine is positive for sugar in dipstick test.
1. **Comment on the diagnosis.**
2. **What are the criteria currently adopted to diagnose diabetes mellitus?**
3. **What other investigations would you like to do in this patient? What is the line of treatment?**

Explanation

This patient is suffering with diabetes. FPG ≥126 mg/dL or HbA1c value of ≥6.5% is one of the criteria for diagnosing diabetes.

The International Expert Committee with the members appointed by ADA, European Association for the Study of Diabetes, and the IDF have issued following **diagnostic criteria for diagnosis of diabetes**:
1. HbA1c ≥6.5%, or
2. FPG ≥126 mg/dL, or

3. 2-hour postprandial plasma glucose ≥200 mg/dL after OGTT (75 g of anhydrous glucose dissolved in water), or
4. Random blood glucose ≥200 mg/dL along with the symptoms of diabetes mellitus.

Most reliable and convenient test is HbA1c or FPG level assessment.

Patient should be thoroughly worked out to rule out diabetic complication. Urine should be investigated for microalbuminuria to rule out impending danger of diabetic nephropathy. Lipid profile should be done, as diabetic patients are prone for dyslipidemia. Patient should be advised oral hypoglycemic treatment along with dietary advice and physical exercise.

Case: Diabetic Ketoacidosis

A 14-year-old boy was admitted in state of coma. His breath was giving fruity odor. He was a known diabetic for 5 years on irregular insulin treatment.

Blood investigation report is as follows:
- Pulse rate: 115/min
- Blood glucose: 408 mg/dL (random)
- BP: 90/60 mm Hg
- pH: 7.05

Urine:
- Protein: Nil
- Ketone bodies: ++++
- Sugar: ++++

1. What is the probable diagnosis?
2. Biochemical basis of the sign and symptoms?
3. What test will you do to find out presence of ketone body in the urine?

Explanation

This boy is having diabetic ketoacidosis characterized by ketone body in body fluid (urine) and in breath. Fruity odor of the breath is due to loss of acetone in the breath.

Rothera's test can be done in the urine to find out ketone body (acetone and acetoacetic acid).

Lack of insulin results in excessive mobilization of fatty acid from adipose cell and its oxidation results in ketoacidosis.

Case: Glucose-6-Phosphate Dehydrogenase Deficiency

A 23-year-old African boy was brought with history of fever and chills and rigors for which he was given antimalarial drug primaquine. Fever subsided but the patient was fatigued with breathlessness. Presently, he is presenting with mild yellow discoloration of conjunctiva. On examination, skin and mucous membrane were pale.
- Hb: 7 gm%
- Total bilirubin: 4 mg%
- Direct bilirubin: 1 mg%
- Indirect bilirubin: 3 mg%
- Fouchet's test: Negative

Liver enzymes are normal.
1. How do you explain this clinical case?

Explanation

Patient may be suffering with G6PD (glucose-6-phosphate dehydrogenase) deficiency. In deficiency of this enzyme, HMP shunt pathway is not able to generate NADPH exposing cells and specifically RBCs for oxidative stress and hemolysis. Treatment with primaquine increases oxidative stress in the cell which causes hemolysis. Patient is presenting with juandice which is due to hemolysis (hemolytic juandice).

Case: Lactose Intolerance

A 2-month-old baby presented to hospital with complain of swelling abdomen and pain after taking milk. Baby is totally alright when fruit juice is given.
1. What is the most probable diagnosis?
2. What is the enzyme deficiency in this case?

Explanation

This baby is suffering with lactose intolerance. This is due to deficiency of **'lactase'** enzyme in intestinal mucosa which results in no digestion of lactose to glucose and galactose. The undigested and unabsorbed lactose in the lumen then becomes a substrate for action of intestinal bacteria which converts lactose to various gases including CO_2 and methane.

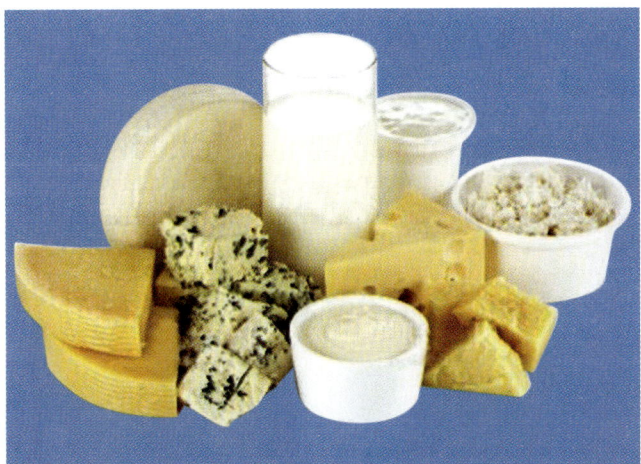

Fig. 24.2: Diet containing rich amount of lactose and galactose

This results in distension and flatulence after consumption of dairy products. Mother is advised to give lactose and galactose-free diet to this baby. Figure 24.2 represents lactose and galactose containing food which should be avoided not only in children suffering with lactose intolerance but also those children who are suffering with galactosemia.

Notes

CHAPTER

25

Interpretation of Laboratory Result: Oral Glucose Tolerance Test (OGTT)

> **Competency**
>
> **BI 3.10:** Interpret the results of blood glucose levels and other laboratory investigations related to disorders of carbohydrate metabolism.

As the name implies, OGTT is the test which evaluates an individual's capability to metabolize glucose load under standard condition and is being tested by serial measurement of blood glucose supplemented with urine examination for glucose.

Following are the recommendations as and when this test needs to be done.

Indications of OGTT
1. To diagnose gestational diabetes mellitus (GDM)
2. Postpartum screening of women for type 2 diabetes mellitus who had GDM.
3. To diagnose impaired glucose tolerance
4. In patients with unexplained neuropathy, nephropathy, retinopathy with RBS <140 mg/dL
5. As a part of epidemiological study

Following are the standard conditions under which this test should be performed:
1. Patient should take at least 150 g of carbohydrate per day for three days prior to test.
2. Test should ideally be done between 7 and 9 am.
3. Patient should be fasting for 10–16 hours.
4. Patient should be ambulatory.
5. Patient should refrain from smoking on the day of testing.

Procedure of the Test
1. After collecting fasting blood and urine, 75 g of anhydrous glucose which is dissolved in 300 mL of water is given to the patient to drink over a period of 5 minutes.
2. Thereafter, blood and urine samples are collected every ½ an hour till 2 hours (total 4 such samples after giving the glucose: ½ hr, 1 hr, 1.5 hr, 2 hr).
3. Plasma glucose in all five samples (including fasting sample) is assessed and urine is checked for presence or absence of glucose using dipstick.
4. Graph is plotted with the values of plasma glucose obtained and result is interpreted.

Interpretation of OGTT Curve Under Various Conditions

To learn the interpretation of OGTT curve, it is important that learner should be familiar with following **WHO criteria** for health and disease and also **ADA criteria** for diagnosis of diabetes (Tables 25.1 and 25.2).

Table 25.1: American Diabetes Association (ADA) diagnostic criteria for diabetes		
Test	Threshold	Qualifier
Hemoglobin A1c or	≥6.5%	Lab NGSP-certified, standardized DCCT assay
Fasting glucose or	≥126 mg/dL (7.0 mmol/L)	No caloric intake for at least 8 hours
2-hour glucose or	≥200 mg/dL (11.1 mmol/L)	After 75 g of anhydrous glucose
Random glucose	≥200 mg/dL (11.1 mmol/L)	Plus classic hyperglycemia symptoms or crisis

NGSP, National Glycohemoglobin Standardization Program; DCCT, Diabetes Control and Complications Trial.
*Results must be confirmed by repeated testing.

Table 25.2: WHO diagnostic criteria for diabetes				
Condition unit	2 hour glucose mmol/L (mg/dL)	Fasting glucose mmol/L (mg/dL)	HbA1c mmol/mol	DCCT%
Normal	<7.8 (<140)	<6.1 (<110)	<42	<6.0
Imparied fasting glycemia	<7.8 (<140)	≥6.1 (≥110) and <7.0 (<126)	42–46	6.0–6.4
Impaired glucose tolerance	≥7.8 (≥140)	<7.0 (<126)	42–46	6.0–6.4
Diabetes mellitus	≥11.1 (≥200)	≥7.0 (≥126)	≥48	≥6.5

OGTT Lab Report Interpretation

Case 1: Following are the OGTT results of a 46-year-old male (Table 25.3).

Table 25.3: OGTT results of a 46-year-old male		
Time (in min)	Plasma glucose (mg/dL)	Urine sugar (Benedict's test)
Fasting	79	Nil
30 (1/2 hr)	118	Nil
60 (1 hr)	140	Nil
90 (1.5 hr)	122	Nil
120 (2 hr)	90	Nil

Q. Interpret the finding.

Result interpretation: The results shown in Table 25.3 and Graph 25.1 represent the 'Normal curve' as in a normal curve, fasting blood glucose is less than 110 mg/dL and it rises to peak (less than 160 mg/dL) at one hour and return to near fasting level (<140 mg/dL) by 2 hours.

Interpretation of Laboratory Result: Oral Glucose Tolerance Test (OGTT)

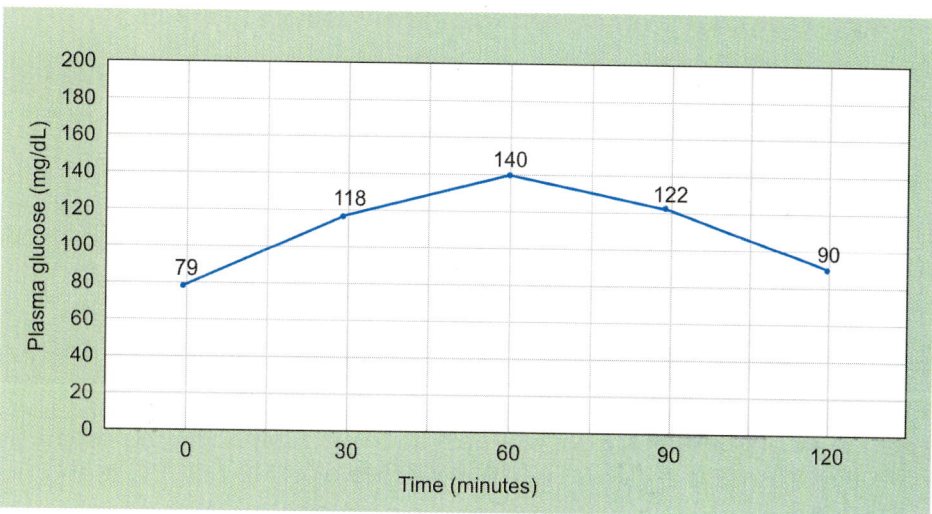

Graph 25.1: Normal OGTT curve

Case 2: Following are the OGTT results of a 55-year-old male (Table 25.4).

Table 25.4: OGTT results of a 55-year-old male		
Time (in min)	Plasma glucose (mg/dL)	Urine sugar (Benedict's test)
Fasting	148	Nil
30 (1/2 hr)	175	Nil
60 (1 hr)	250	++
90 (1.5 hr)	240	++
120 (2 hr)	210	+

Q. Interpret the finding.
Result interpretation: The results shown in Table 25.4 and Graph 25.2 represent the diabetes mellitus as FPG is >126 mg/dL and 2-hour postprandial value of plasma glucose is >200 mg/dL.

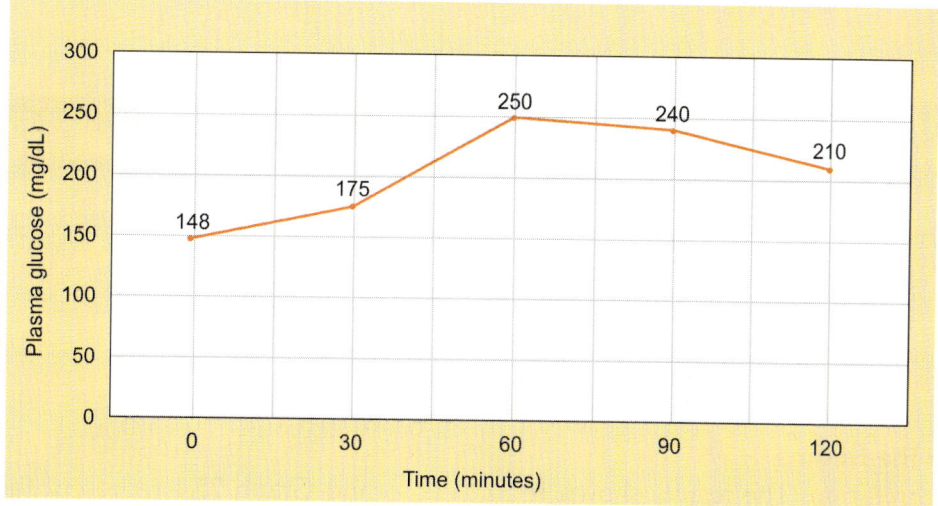

Graph 25.2: OGTT curve in diabetes mellitus

Case 3: Following are the OGTT results of a 62-year-old female (Table 25.5).

Table 25.5: OGTT results of a 62-year-old female		
Time (in min)	Plasma glucose (mg/dL)	Urine sugar (Benedict's test)
Fasting	114	Nil
30 (1/2 hr)	120	Nil
60 (1 hr)	122	Nil
90 (1.5 hr)	135	Nil
120 (2 hr)	138	Nil

Q. Interpret the finding.

Result interpretation: The results shown in Table 25.5 and Graph 25.3 represent the impaired fasting glycemia curve as fasting glucose is 114 mg% (between 110 and 125 mg%).

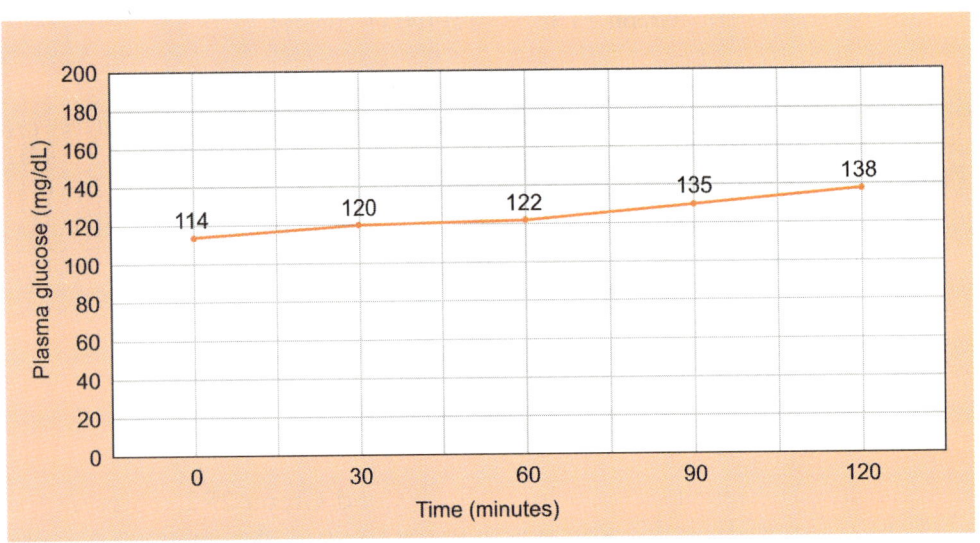

Graph 25.3: OGTT curve in impaired fasting glycemia

Case 4: Following are the OGTT results of a 54-year-old male (Table 25.6).

Table 25.6: OGTT results of a 54-year-old male		
Time (in min)	Plasma glucose (mg/dL)	Urine sugar (Benedict's test)
Fasting	95	Nil
30 (1/2 hr)	110	Nil
60 (1 hr)	130	Nil
90 (1.5 hr)	140	Nil
120 (2 hr)	185	+

Q. Interpret the finding.

Result interpretation: The results shown in Table 25.6 and Graph 25.4 represent the impaired glucose tolerance curve. Here 2-hour plasma glucose value is 185 mg% (>140 to <200 mg%).

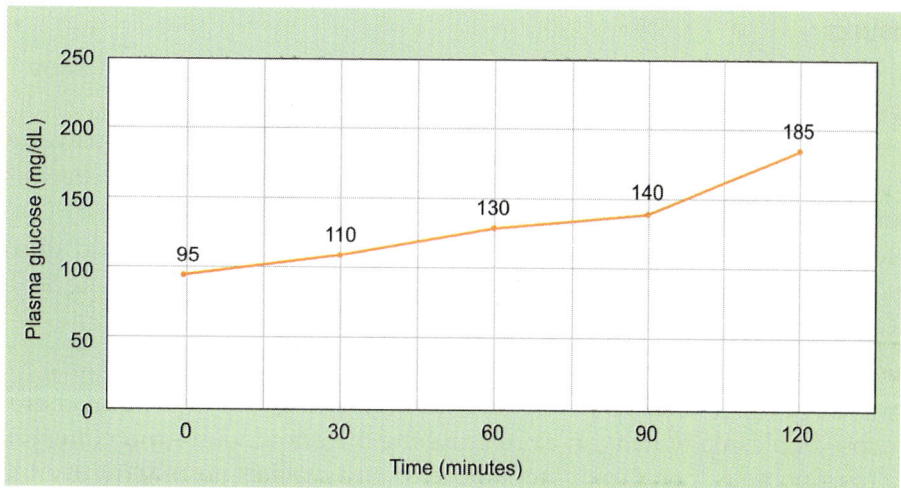

Graph 25.4: OGTT curve of impaired glucose tolerance curve

Case 5: Following are the OGTT results of a 66-year-old female (Table 25.7).

Table 25.7: OGTT results of a 66-year-old female		
Time (in min)	Plasma glucose (mg/dL)	Urine sugar (Benedict's test)
Fasting	90	Nil
30 (1/2 hr)	120	++
60 (1 hr)	125	++
90 (1.5 hr)	100	Nil
120 (2 hr)	95	Nil

Q. Interpret the finding.

Result interpretation: The results shown in Table 25.7 and Graph 25.5 represent the state of renal glycosuria.

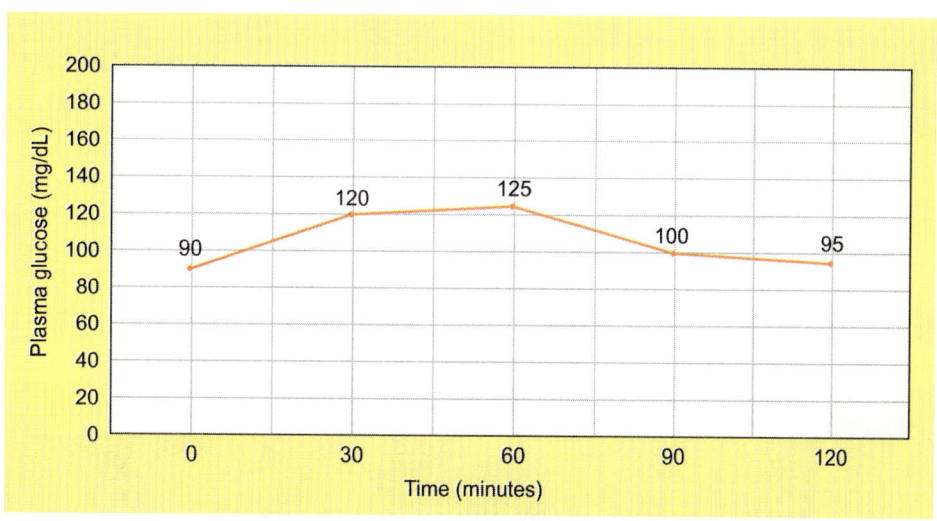

Graph 25.5: OGTT curve of renal glycosuria

Renal Glycosuria

Normal **renal threshold for glucose is 180 mg/dL**, it means that urine will show glucose only when blood glucose value raises above 180 mg/dL.

In case of renal glycosuria, glucose appears in the urine even at lower plasma values of glucose.

This is occasionally seen in third trimester of pregnancy and sometimes in harmless situations of reabsorption defect in kidney tubules.

[Contrary to above situation, at times the renal threshold is increased and glucose does not appear in the urine even when the level of plasma glucose raises beyond 180 mg %. This is seen in case of **glomerular arteriosclerosis** in elderly patients with diabetes.]

Case 6: Alimentary glycosuria (lag curve)

In this case, there is exaggerated response to glucose loading and at 1 hour, there is very high amount of glucose in plasma which can even cross the threshold value and come out in the urine (glycosuria). This glucose is then rapidly metabolized and reaches normal (or even hypoglycemic level occasionally) by the end of two hours.

This is due to rapid emptying of stomach in cases of hyperthyroidism and partial gastrectomy. It is also called lag curve on assumption that there is lag in insulin secretion resulting in high glucose levels at 1-hour period.

It is a harmless condition and does not need any active intervention.

Following may be the finding in OGTT in a patient having alimentary glycosuria (Table 25.8 and Graph 25.6).

Table 25.8: OGTT in a patient having alimentary glycosuria		
Time (in min)	Plasma glucose (mg/dL)	Urine sugar (Benedict's test)
Fasting	79	Nil
30 (1/2 hr)	118	Nil
60 (1 hr)	**198**	+
90 (1.5 hr)	122	Nil
120 (2 hr)	60	Nil

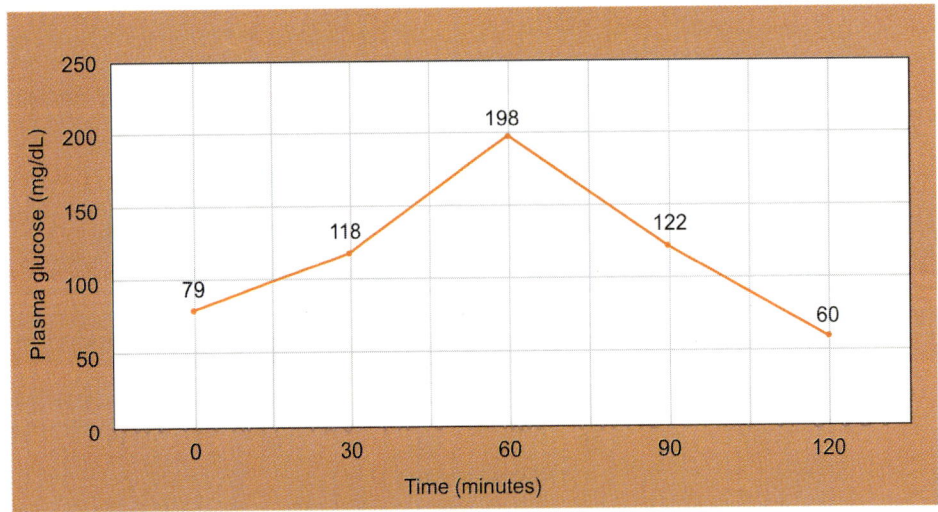

Graph 25.6: OGTT curve in alimentary glycosuria [lag curve]

Case 7: Following may be the finding in OGTT in a patient showing increased glucose tolerance (Table 25.9 and Graph 25.7).

Table 25.9: OGTT in a patient showing increased glucose tolerance		
Time (in min)	Plasma glucose (mg/dL)	Urine sugar (Benedict's test)
Fasting	79	Nil
30 (1/2 hr)	81	Nil
60 (1 hr)	**84**	**Nil**
90 (1.5 hr)	80	Nil
120 (2 hr)	78	Nil

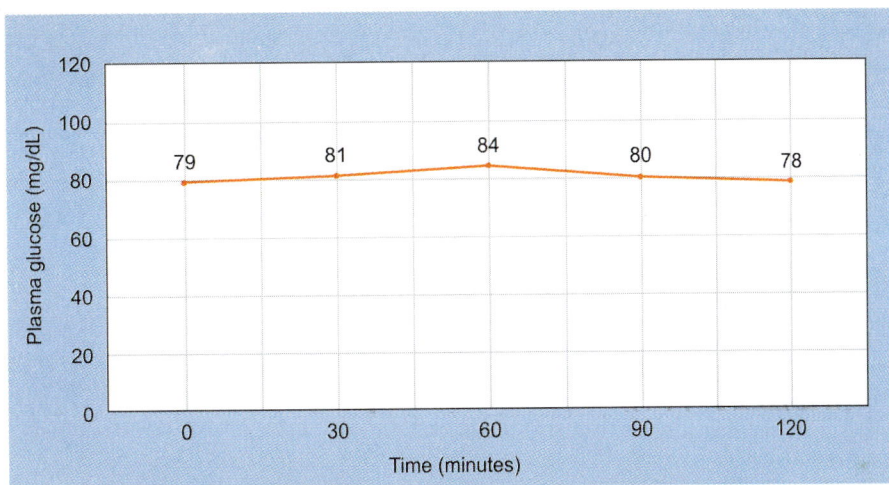

Graph 25.7: Flat curve [increased glucose tolerance curve]

Flat curve (increased glucose tolerance curve): In this, patient shows little or no effect of glucose loading on blood glucose. Even at 1 hr, the level of plasma glucose remains near fasting values which again is within normal limits.

This is due to malabsorption, hypothyroidism, hypopituitarism, hypoadrenalism.

OGTT in Pregnancy to Rule Out Gestational Diabetes Mellitus (GDM)

It is done in high-risk pregnant women who have family history of diabetes or history of diabetes in previous pregnancy or advanced maternal age.

It is done with **100 grams of anhydrous glucose**.

Following are considered upper normal limit (Table 25.10).

Table 25.10: OGTT in pregnancy (GDM)	
Sample collection time	Value of glucose (mg/dL)
Fasting	105
1 hr	190
2 hr	165
3 hr	145

If any of two values exceeds the above values given in Table 25.10 is suggestive of gestational diabetes mellitus (GDM).

Notes

CHAPTER

26

Interpretation of Laboratory Result: Amino Acid Metabolism

Competency

BI 5.5: Interpret laboratory results of analytes associated with metabolism of amino acid.

Urea Cycle Disorder

A 2-year-old male baby is presented with history of aversion to protein-containing food and frequent episode of vomiting. On examination, baby was lethargic and mentally retarded.

Blood showed high level of ammonia and urine examination denotes presence of orotic acid. Diagnosis of urea cycle disorder was made.

What may be the most probable enzyme deficiency in this baby?

Explanation

Ornithine transcarboxylase (OTC) deficiency is the most common cause of urea cycle disorder. It is an X-linked disorder and males are more seriously affected than heterozygous female.

Orotic acid is produced in excess amount due to no utilization of carbamoyl phosphate in urea cycle and its diffusion to the cytosol where it is diverted to pyrimidine nucleotide biosynthesis.

Mental retardation is due to excess ammonia and delay in treatment.

Maple Syrup Urine Disease (MSUD)

A five-month-old female child presenting with fits and refusal to feed. Baby was normal at birth and her condition progressively deteriorated over five days. Urine of the baby gave characteristic burnt sugar odor.

DNPH (dinitrophenyl hydrazine) test performed on urine gave yellow white precipitate (Fig. 26.1) and ferric chloride test gave greyish blue color. Diagnosis of maple syrup urine disease was made.

Comment of clinical condition baby is suffering from.

Explanation

MSUD is also known as branched chain ketoaciduria (oxoaciduria). It is an autosomal recessive disorder. Enzyme which is deficient is "branched chain alpha-ketoacid dehydrogenase complex" (BCKD)/also known as decarboxylase. This is the second enzyme during branched chain amino acid catabolism. Mutation may be on any of the gene encoding enzyme E1, E2 or E3 of the enzyme

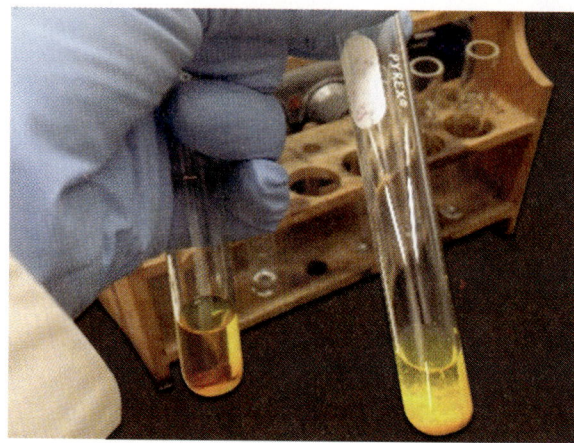

Fig. 26.1: DNPH test for MSUD

complex and disease presents with different severity depending upon the extent of deficiency of these enzymes.

Child is normal at birth but neurological deterioration is observed in first 3 to 4 days of birth when they present with apnea, seizures and death. If they survive, severe mental retardation is inevitable.

Fresh urine has characteristic **'odor'** of maple syrup (boiled Chinese herb). [Picture of maple syrup and its plant is shown in Fig. 26.2; please note that it is the odor and not the color of urine which is similar to maple syrup.]

Treatment is giving formula diet (Fig. 26.3) where restriction of branched chain amino acid specially leucine is done.

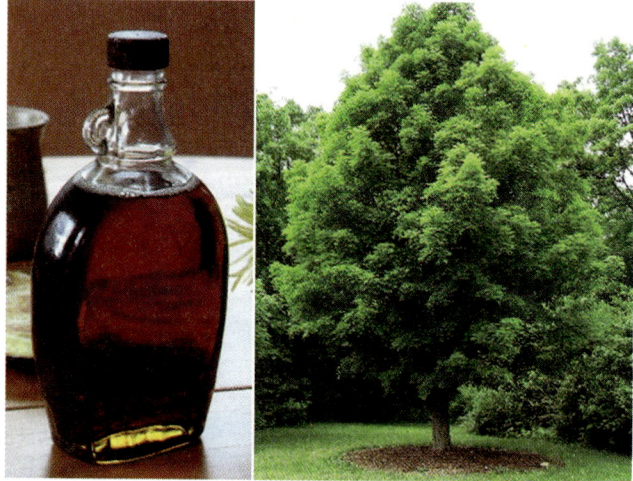

Fig. 26.2: Maple syrup and its plant

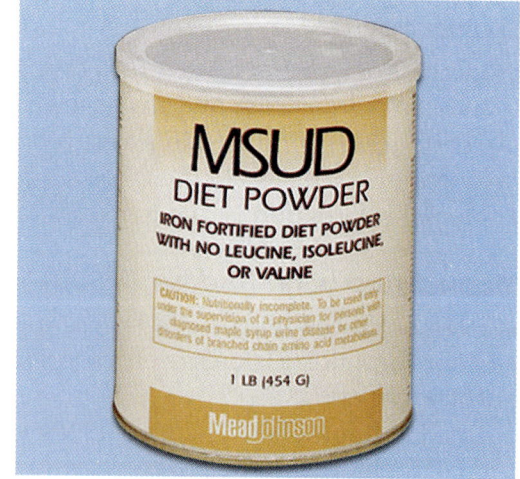

Fig. 26.3: Formula diet in MSUD

Classical or Typical Homocystinuria

A 4-year-old child from poor socioeconomic background presents with low IQ, defective vision, skeletal deformity (genu valgum, osteoporosis, vertebral anomaly). Cardiovascular system involvement is seen, and lens was showing dislocation (ectopia lentis). Child had myopia (near sightedness).
Comment on the probable diagnosis.

Explanation

This child is suffering with homocystinuria which is due to defect in methionine amino acid metabolism. It is of following subtypes:

a. Type I (Typical/Classical): Due to deficiency of 'cystathionine beta-synthase'.
b. Type II: Due to deficiency of N5, N10-Methylenetetrahydrofolate reductase.
c. Type III: Due to deficiency of homocysteine methyltransferase.
d. Type IV: Due to deficiency of vitamin B_{12} (associated with methyl malonic acidemia).

Typical Homocystinuria

- It is autosomal recessive disorder due to deficiency of enzyme 'cystathionine beta-synthase' which is dependent on vitamin B_6.
- Clinical manifestations in typical homocystinuria involve following organ systems (Fig. 26.4):
  - **Eye** (subluxation of lens, secondary glaucoma, optic atrophy, retinal detachment)
  - **Central nervous system** (cerebellar ataxia, nystagmus, aphasia, hypotonia and muscle weakness)
  - **Vascular** (thromboembolic episodes and atherosclerosis)
  - **Skeleton** (arachnodactyly, lengthening of long bones, osteoporosis, scoliosis).
- Mild to moderate degree of mental retardation is seen in 50 to 75% of patients.
- Treatment is restriction of protein and methionine. Vitamin B_6 supplementation may help as it may increase residual activity of cystathionine beta-synthase. Supplementation of betaine, vitamin B_{12} (hydroxocobalamin), methyl tetrahydrofolate also to be done.

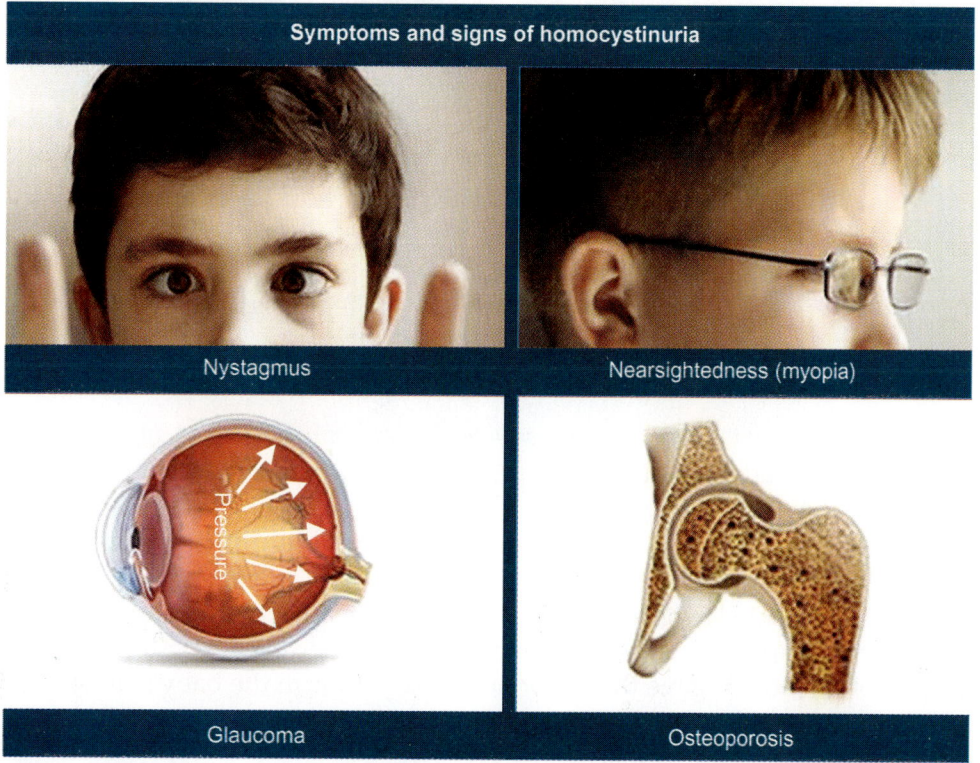

Fig. 26.4: Findings in a case of homocystinuria—clockwise: 1. Nystagmus; 2. Myopia; 3. Osteoporosis; 4. Glaucoma

Alkaptonuria

A 12-year-old child is presenting with complain of back pain and knee pain. Urine turns black after a few hours of exposure to atmospheric oxygen. His ear pinnae show black pigmentation.
Comment on the clinical condition this patient may be suffering from.

Explanation

This boy has typical presentation of alkaptonuria.

Alkaptonuria is an autosomal recessive disorder which is due to deficiency of enzyme homogentisic acid oxidase (HGA oxidase), involved in phenylalanine and tyrosine catabolism. In deficiency of this enzyme, homogentisic acid (HGA) is not further metabolized.

HGA is a colorless substance which is excreted in urine and undergo auto-oxidation to corresponding quinone. These quinones undergo polymerization to blackish pigment 'Alkapton' which imparts black color to urine. Fresh urine is colorless but on exposure to atmospheric oxygen urine turns black.

HGA also gets deposited in articular cartilages of knee, hip and shoulder and resulting in arthritis of these joints. Intervertebral disc also is the site where such deposit results in backpain. Deposition of these pigments can be visualized in ear pinnae. Deposition of these pigments in these tissues is termed as **'ochronosis'** due to Ochre color of the deposits (Fig. 26.5).

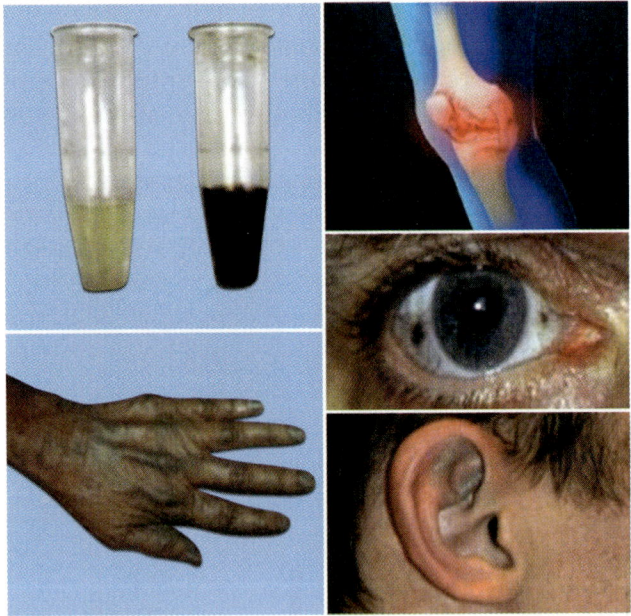

Fig. 26.5: Clockwise: Black urine, arthritis, black pigment deposit in sclera, ear pinnae and dorsum hand in a typical case of alkaptonuria

Phenylketonuria

A 6-month-old child presented to hospital with history of generalized fits. Baby was born by normal delivery without forceps application. On examination, baby had delayed milestone and was lethargic, hair was grey colored, mother gave the history of mousy odor in the baby skin, hair and urine.
1. **What is the most probable diagnosis in this case?**
2. **What test is done to confirm the diagnosis?**
3. **What treatment is advised for this baby?**
4. **Why the baby hair is grey?**

Explanation

This baby is suffering with phenylketonuria (PKU) which is due to defect in enzyme/s responsible for conversion of phenylalanine to tyrosine. The most common enzyme deficient in PKU is **phenylalanine hydroxylase**. Other enzymes which may be deficient are **DHB reductase** and **DHB synthase** (Fig. 26.6). In alternate pathway, phenylalanine is converted to phenylketones which cause impaired neurological development and mental retardation.

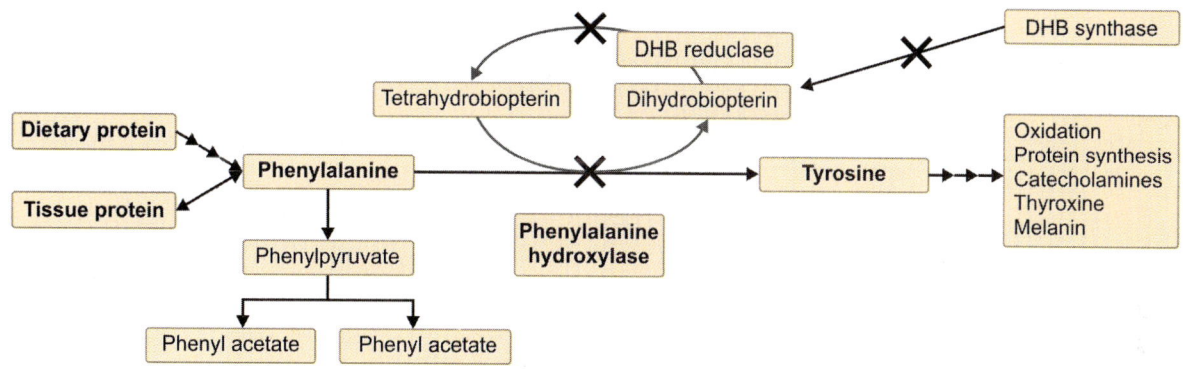

Fig. 26.6: Biochemical pathway involved in phenylketonuria (PKU)

Tyrosine is the precursor amino acid for synthesis of melanin. In phenylketonuria, due to lack of synthesis of tyrosine from phenylalanine, melanin synthesis does not take place resulting in greying of hair. In addition, phenylalanine is a competitive inhibitor of tyrosinase enzyme which is required for melanin synthesis.

Urine has characteristic mousy or musty odor which is due to phenylacetate component. Screening can be done by **ferric chloride test** of the urine which gives leafy green color as positive test. Confirmation is done by **Guthrie test** in the blood of the patient.

Dietary treatment is advised where restriction of phenylalanine and supplementation of tyrosine is done lifelong.

Albinism

A 14-year-old female is presenting to ophthalmology OPD for eye check-up as she is having photophobia and discomfort in eye. Her skin and hair are white (Fig. 26.7).

What is the biochemical defect in this case?

Explanation

This girl is suffering with albinism which is due to mutation of tyrosinase gene. Tyrosinase is the enzyme needed for synthesis of melanin. Melanin is a pigment which is responsible for black pigmentation of hair and skin.

It is an autosomal recessive disorder with the incidence of 1/20,000 population.

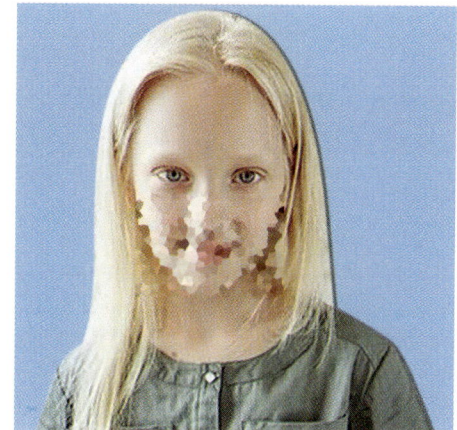

Fig. 26.7: Albinism

Skin is pinkish white and hair is brown. Nystagmus, poor vision and photophobia are commonly associated.

Notes

CHAPTER

27

Interpretation of Laboratory Result: Lipid Metabolism

> **Competencies**

BI 4.5, BI 4.7, IM 2.12: Discussion on certain lab reports related to lipid profile.
BI 11.17: Tests done to find out the dyslipidemia and its type and the rationale behind it.

Following are the list of tests which are being done under lipid profile in a case of dyslipidemia:
- Total cholesterol
- HDL cholesterol
- LDL cholesterol
- Triglyceride
- VLDL
- Apo B
- Apo A
- LDL/HDL ratio
- TC/HDL ratio
- Lipoprotein (a)

Normal lipid profile of adult is enlisted in Table 27.1.

Lab report 1: Following is the lipid profile of a 42-year-old patient who presents with complain of yellow nodular deposition around the eye for past 6 months (Fig. 27.1).
- Total cholesterol: 380 mg/dL
- HDL cholesterol: 35 mg/dL
- LDL cholesterol: 317 mg/dL
- Triglyceride: 140 mg/dL
- VLDL: 28 mg/dL

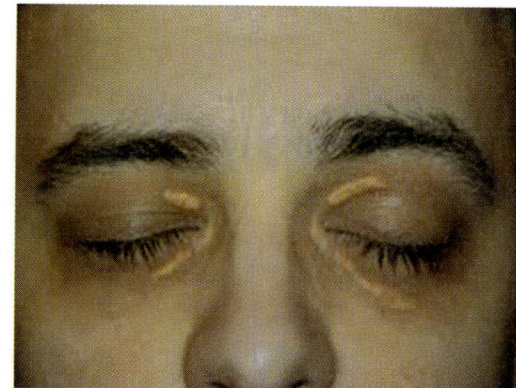

Fig. 27.1: Xanthelasma

What is the interpretation?

Ans: This patient is suffering with type IIa hyperlipoproteinemia (familial hypercholesterolemia). In this disease, the clearance of LDL is affected either because of mutation of LDL receptor at hepatocyte or due to mutation of ApoB100 of LDL particle.

This disease is characterized by tendon xanthomas, xanthelasma and vascular disease.

Table 27.1: Values of various lipid parameters in a healthy adult	
Parameters	Normal healthy adult
Total cholesterol	Desirable: <200 mg/dL Borderline high: 200 to 239 mg/dL High: >240 mg/dL
HDL cholesterol	40–75 mg/dL
LDL cholesterol	Optimal: <100 mg/dL Near optimal: 100 to 129 mg/dL Borderline high: 130 to 159 mg/dL High: 160 to 189 mg/dL Very high: >190 mg/dL
Triglyceride	60–150 mg/dL
VLDL	<40 mg/dL
Free fatty acid	200–800 µmol/L
Lipoprotein (a)	0 to 30 mg/dL

Heterozygous state is more prevalent (1: 500) and manifestation is seen in adults only. Homozygous state is less prevalent (1: 1 million) and manifestation is seen in childhood.

Lab report 2: Following is the lipid profile result of a patient who presents with acute pancreatitis:
- Total cholesterol: 194 mg/dL
- HDL cholesterol: 32 mg/dL
- LDL cholesterol: 92 mg/dL
- Triglyceride: 350 mg/dL
- VLDL: 70 mg/dL

Ans: Patient is suffering with isolated hypertriacylglyceridemia [type I (familial hypertriacylglyceridemia) or type V hyperlipoproteinemia]. In type I hyperlipidemia, there is lack of lipoprotein lipase enzyme and in type V hyperlipidemia there is deficiency of apo C. Both these conditions result in lack of activity of lipoprotein lipase enzyme which is reflected in elevation of VLDL and chylomicron.

This condition may be asymptomatic or may present with pancreatitis as in this case.

Lab report 3: A 46-year-old patient with history of heart disease is presenting with following lipid profile. Interpret the finding.
- Total cholesterol: 345 mg/dL
- HDL cholesterol: 42 mg/dL
- LDL cholesterol: 233 mg/dL
- Triglyceride: 350 mg/dL
- VLDL: 70 mg/dL

Ans: Patient is suffering with **type IIb hyperlipoproteinemia (familial combined hyperlipidemia)** which is due to impaired clearance of LDL from the plasma and in addition excessive secretion of VLDL from liver.

Patient has high level of LDL cholesterol and as the major contribution of total cholesterol is from the LDL, total cholesterol is also high in such patients. Triacylglycerol level is also high due to excessive VLDL secretion from liver.

Lab report 4: Following is the lipid profile report in otherwise healthy 43-year-old male. Comment on the condition.
- Total cholesterol: 240 mg/dL
- HDL cholesterol: 45 mg/dL
- LDL cholesterol: 145 mg/dL
- Triglyceride: 250 mg/dL
- VLDL: 50 mg/dL
- Lipoprotein electrophoresis shows 'broad beta band'

Ans: Patient is having **type III hyperlipoproteinemia** or **remnant removal disease (familial dysbetalipoproteinemia)**. This condition is mostly asymptomatic till vascular disease develops. Palmar or tuberous xanthomas may be found.

Lab report 5: Following is the lipid profile report in otherwise healthy 50-year-old male suffering with diabetes. Comment on the condition.
- Total cholesterol: 190 mg/dL
- HDL cholesterol: 45 mg/dL
- LDL cholesterol: 75 mg/dL
- Triglyceride: 350 mg/dL
- VLDL: 70 mg/dL

Ans: Patient is suffering with type IV hyperlipoproteinemia.

This is due to excessive VLDL secretion from liver due to idiopathic cause. This condition may be asymptomatic or may be associated with vascular features.

Friedewald Equation

It is commonly used indirect method of LDL assessment. Total cholesterol, HDL cholesterol, triglyceride measurement is done and LDL is calculated using following formula:

$$LDL = [Total\ cholesterol] - [HDL\ cholesterol] - [TAG/5]$$

TAG/5 represents the level of VLDL cholesterol. This is because the average ratio of TAG to the cholesterol in the VLDL is five, which means TAG is almost five times to that of cholesterol in the VLDL.

Friedewald equation cannot be applied in following conditions:
1. Samples where TAG concentration is >400 mg/dL.
2. Non-fasting sample where chylomicron is also there in plasma which alters the value of TAG.
3. Type III hyperlipoproteinemia (due to abnormal VLDL composition where TAG/5 cannot be applied).

Notes

CHAPTER 28

Interpretation of Laboratory Result: Protein Metabolism

> **Competency**
>
> **BI 5.5:** Interpret laboratory results of analytes associated with metabolism of proteins.

Following case report will be described under this heading:
1. Kwashiorkor
2. Marasmus
3. Nephrotic syndrome
4. Alcoholic liver cirrhosis
5. Multiple myeloma

Kwashiorkor

A 4-year-old child of poor socioeconomic strata presents with the history of weakness, lethargy and swelling all over the body. On examination, he was found to have pitting pedal edema, marked muscle atrophy, distension of abdomen along with hepatomegaly (Fig. 28.1).

Following were the biochemical findings:
- Total protein: 4.5 g/dL (N = 6.5–8 g/dL)
- Albumin: 1.5 g/dL (N = 4–6 g/dL)
- Blood glucose: 98 mg/dL (normal random blood glucose: 90 to 140 mg/dL)
- Total cholesterol 90 mg/dL (desirable < 200 mg/dL)

1. What may be the diagnosis in this case?
2. What will be the treatment in this case?

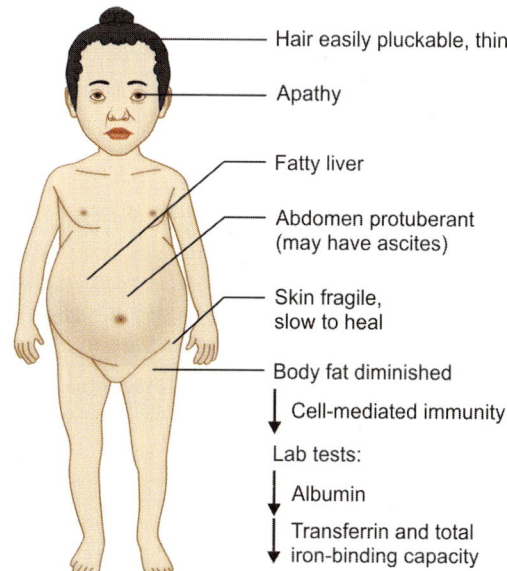

Fig. 28.1: Representation of a child showing features of kwashiorkor

Explanation

This baby is suffering with **Kwashiorkor**, a disease which is due to adequate calorie intake but lack of protein in the diet. Kwashiorkor is a disease characterized by bilateral extremity swelling, round facies (moon facies) and protruded abdomen. Marked muscle atrophy is noticed.

It usually affects infants and children, most often around the age of weaning through age of five years. Diets based mainly on maize, cassava, or rice are frequently associated with the disease. Pedal edema results from a loss of fluid balance between hydrostatic and oncotic pressures across capillary blood vessel walls. Albumin contributes to the oncotic pressure, allowing the fluid to be retained within the vasculature. Children with kwashiorkor are found to have profoundly low levels of albumin and, as a result, become intravascularly depleted.

Marasmus

A one-year-old child of poor socioeconomic strata presents with prominent rib cage, severe loss of weight, lethargy, shrunken eye (Fig. 28.2). On examination child was emaciated. Eyes were pale and muscle hypotonia was present.

Lab findings:
- Total protein: 6 g/dL
- Albumin: 3 g/dL
- Blood glucose: 67 mg/dL

1. What is the suffering of child?
2. What are the key differences in marasmus and kwashiorkor?

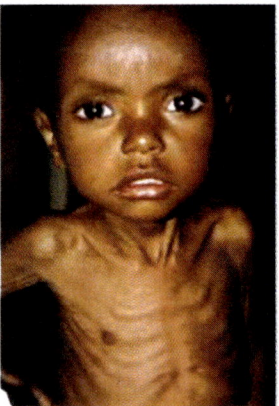

Fig. 28.2: A child suffering with marasmus

Explanation

This child is suffering with severe form of malnutrition which is due to lack of both carbohydrate and protein in the diet. Marasmus is the most prevalent form of malnutrition in developing country like India. It is an important cause of child mortality rate in our country. This is because of insufficient food intake because of poverty and no availability of food. Deficiencies of minerals and vitamins are also associated.

Superimposed parasitic infection exaggerates the deficiency by impairing the absorption and assimilation of nutrients. Child presents with impaired physical growth, and inadequate social and economic development.

Key Differences in Marasmus and Kwashiorkor

Kwashiorkor	Marasmus
It develops in children whose diet is deficient in protein with adequate carbohydrate intake	It is due to deficiency of proteins and carbohydrate both in the diet
It occurs in children between 6 months and 3 years of age	It is common in infants under 1 year of age
Subcutaneous fat is preserved	Subcutaneous fat is not preserved
Edema is present	Edema is absent
Enlarged fatty liver	No fatty liver
Ribs are not very prominent	Ribs become very prominent
Lethargic	Alert and irritable
Muscle wasting mild or absent	Severe muscle wasting
Poor appetite	Varacious feeder
The person suffering from Kwashiorkor needs adequate amounts of proteints	The person suffering from Marasmus needs adequate amount of protein, fats and carbohydrates.

Nephrotic Syndrome

A 4-year-old male child is admitted with the history of recurrent episode of puffiness of the face (which is more prominent in the morning), generalized weakness and loss of appetite.

Following were the results of urine and blood investigations.

Blood:
- Total protein: 4.9 g/dL (N= 6.5–8 g/dL)
- Albumin: 2.5 g/dL (N = 4–6 g/dL)
- Globulin: 2.4 g/dL (1.5 to 3.5 g/dL)
- Total cholesterol 450 mg/dL (desirable <200 mg/dL)
- Blood urea: 97 mg/dL (10–40 mg/dL)
- Serum creatinine: 1.8 mg/dL (<1 mg/dL)

Urine: Total protein in 24-hour urine collection: 4.5 g (normal protein excretion in urine <150 mg/dL).

1. **Comment on the diagnosis. What are the diagnostic criteria of nephrotic syndrome?**
2. **What is the reason of facial puffiness in this child?**

Explanation

This child is most probably suffering with acute episode of nephrotic syndrome. Nephrotic syndrome is not a disease rather a group of disorders characterized by loss of protein in the urine.

Childhood nephrotic syndrome may be primary or secondary **(Fig. 28.3)**.

1. **Primary childhood nephrotic syndrome** is the most common type which may be due to following pathologies:
a. Minimal change disease
b. Focal segmental glomerulosclerosis
c. Membranoproliferative glomerulonephritis

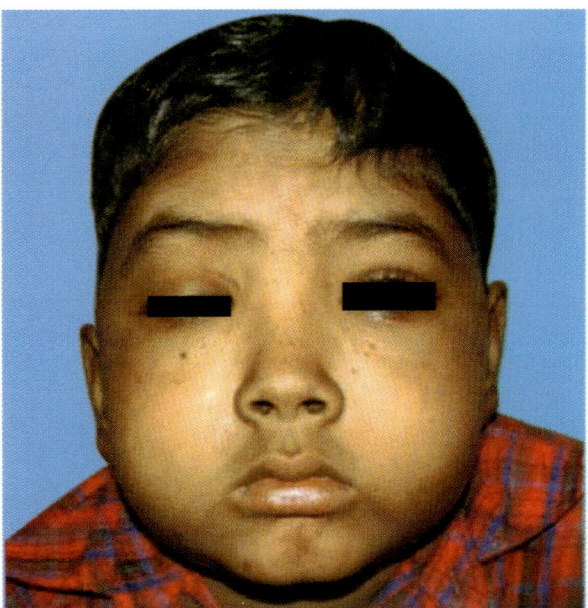

Fig. 28.3: Facial puffiness in a child of nephrotic syndrome

2. **Secondary childhood nephrotic syndrome** is associated with certain other systemic pathology like diabetes, IgA vasculitis, hepatitis, lupus, malaria, HIV, streptococcal infection.

Following are the diagnostic criteria for nephrotic syndrome:
- Proteinuria >3 g/dL
- Hypoalbuminemia
- Hypercholesterolemia
- Edema and hypertension

Facial puffiness is due to loss of albumin from the plasma which results in exudation of fluid from intravascular space.

Alcoholic Liver Cirrhosis

A 49-year-old chronic alcoholic is coming with complain of loss of weight, generalized weakness, nausea, vomiting and pain in right upper quadrant. On examination, patient had ascites and mild hepatomegaly. Yellow discoloration of sclera was noticed. Finger showed clubbing and palmar erythema was noticed (Figs 28.4 and 28.5).

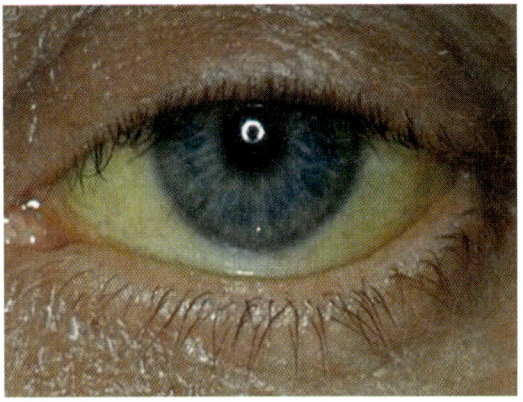

Fig. 28.4: Yellow discoloration of sclera

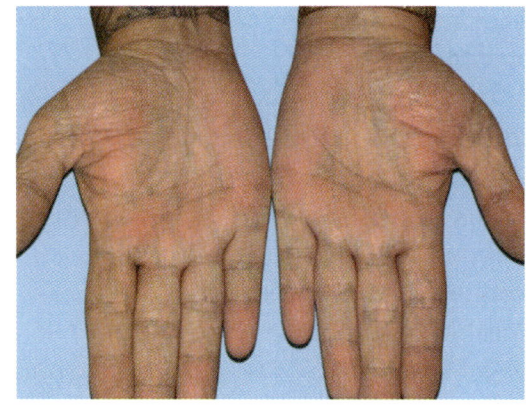

Fig. 28.5: Palmar erythema

Following are the biochemical findings in this patient:
- Total protein: 5.4 g/dL
- Albumin: 3 g/dL
- Total bilirubin: 1.8 mg/dL
- Conjugated bilirubin: 0.8 mg/dL
- Unconjugated bilirubin: 1.0 mg/dL
- AST: 410 IU/L
- ALT: 204 IUL
- AST: ALT ratio is 2:1
- GGT: 370 IU/L
- Prothrombin time: Elevated

Comment on the diagnosis and justify the biochemical finding.

Explanation

This patient is most likely suffering with **alcoholic cirrhosis**, a condition where liver architecture is distorted due to fibrosis which reduces the effective mass of liver and adversely affects the liver function. Liver being the main site for albumin production, the level of plasma albumin is reduced considerably which is manifested in the form of edema and ascites.

Prothrombin time is elevated due to impaired post-translational modification of clotting factors due to liver dysfunction.

Elevation of GGT is characteristic finding seen in alcoholic hepatitis which is because of proliferation of endoplasmic reticulum.

AST:ALT ratio is known as **De Ritis index** and normal ratio is 1:1 considering the equal concentration of AST and ALT in the plasma (30–40 IU/L).

The ratio of 1.5 to 2 is suggestive of alcoholic liver disease. The predominance of AST over ALT in alcohol-related liver disease was first reported by Harinasuta et al in 1967. Many authors since then have described AST/ALT ratios greater than 1.5 or 2.0 as being highly suggestive of alcoholic hepatitis.

(ALT is present in the hepatocyte cytoplasm alone whereas AST is present in hepatocyte cytoplasm and mitochondria both. Cytosolic AST (cAST) and mitochondrial AST (mAST) are true isoenzymes and are immunologically distinct. mAST is the more prevalent isoenzyme with approximately 80% of total AST activity in human liver contributed by mAST.)

Multiple Myeloma

A 57-year-old male who is a labour in leather industry is coming in a state of confusion with complain of generalized bone pain, weakness and numbness of lower limbs for past 6 months. He gives the history of repeated lung infection for past few months. On examination, he was found to be anemic.

Following were the blood investigation reports:
- Serum total calcium: 12 mg/dL
- ALP: 55 IU/L
- Hb: 7 g/dL
- Serum urea: 56 mg/dL
- Serum creatinine: 1.6 mg/dL
- Serum uric acid: 7.8 mg/dL
- Total protein: 7.5 g/dL
- Albumin: 3.0 g/dL
- Globulin: 4.5 g/dL

X-ray skull typically showed **punched out lesion** (Fig. 28.6).

On protein electrophoresis **M band was found** (Fig. 28.7).

Urine shows presence of **Bence Jones protein (BJP)**.

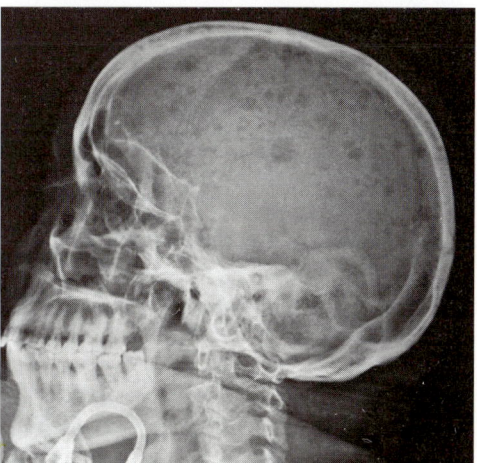

Fig. 28.6: Punched out lesion in multiple myeloma

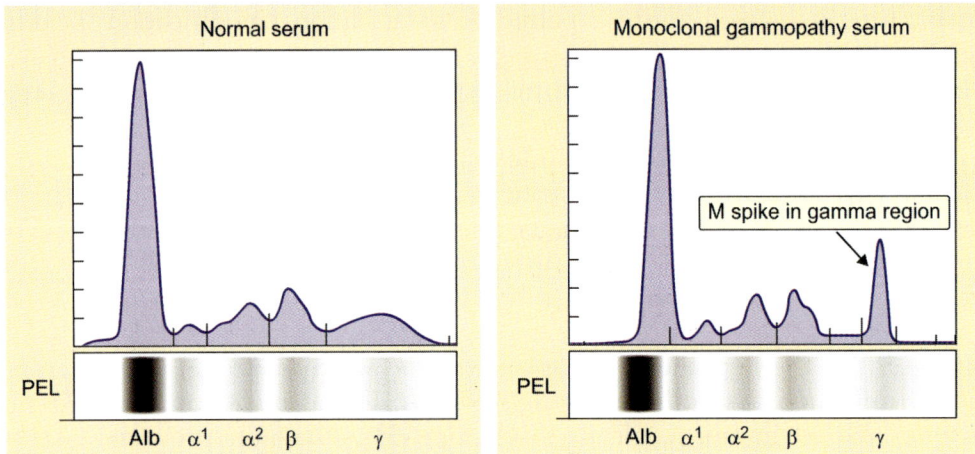

Fig. 28.7: M band on EPP in multiple myeloma

Comment on the diagnosis in this case.

Explanation

This patient is suffering with **multiple myeloma**, which is a **malignant proliferation of plasma cell** derived from single clone. Most commonly these patients present with generalized bone pain and fracture bone and anemia. Susceptibility of infection is common in such patients.

Myeloma cell produces many osteoclastic activating factors which results in osteolytic lesions which may involve even the skull (punched out lytic lesion).

Increased susceptibility to infection is due to diffuse hypogammaglobulinemia.

Anemia is due to replacement of normal marrow by expanding tumour cell, and also because of reduced production of erythropoietin by the kidney.

Notes

CHAPTER

29

Interpretation of Laboratory Result: Purine Nucleotide Metabolism

> **Competency**
>
> **BI 6.4:** Discuss the laboratory results of analytes associated with gout and Lesch-Nyhan syndrome.

Gout

A 47-year-old presenting to the emergency OPD with complain of sudden onset of pain in right wrist joint followed by pain in the left metatarsophalangeal joint (Fig. 29.1). He was indulged in new year party previous night where he consumed liquor along with non-vegetarian diet.

Blood examination revealed:
- Total protein: 6.9 g/dL (N= 6.5–8 g/dL)
- Albumin: 3.9 g/dL (N = 4–6 g/dL)
- Blood urea: 37 mg/dL
- Serum creatinine: 1.0 mg/dL
- Serum uric acid: 8.6 mg/dL

1. What is the probable diagnosis?
2. What may be the link of alcohol consumption and precipitation of this acute attack?
3. What is the confirmatory test for making the diagnosis?

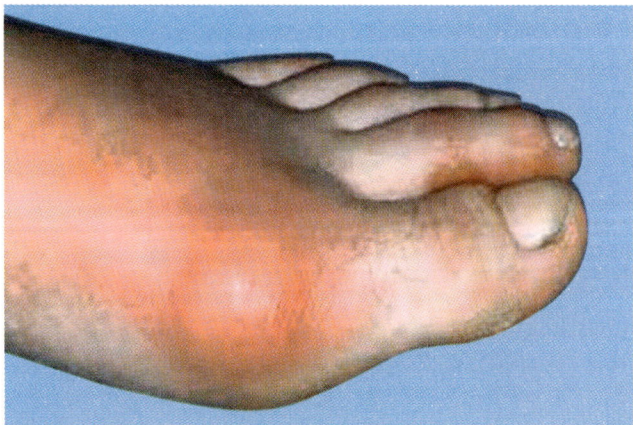

Fig. 29.1: Swelling at metatarsophalangeal joint (big toe) in a case of gout

Explanation

1. This patient may be suffering with acute attack of gout. **Gout** is a metabolic disease characterized by acute or chronic arthritis which is due to deposition of **monosodium urate (MSU) crystals** in joints and soft tissues. Classically described as a disease associated with hyperuricemia which may be due to metabolic defect in uric acid production or due to impaired renal excretion. This disease has strong genetic predisposition and tend to affect elderly men and postmenopausal women more commonly.
2. Alcohol is thought to increase the risk of gout because the metabolism of ethanol to acetyl CoA leads to adenine nucleotide degradation, resulting in increased formation of adenosine monophosphate, a precursor of uric acid. Alcohol metabolism also raises the lactic acid level in blood, which inhibits uric acid excretion.
3. Gold standard of diagnosis is visualization of MSU (monosodium urate) crystals in the synovial fluid. **MSU crystals are negatively birefringent crystals.** They show characteristic color when exposed to plane polarized light. When the axis of the MSU crystal is parallel to the polarizer, it appears **yellow**. When it is perpendicular, it appears **blue** (Fig. 29.2).
4. MSU crystals are found in synovial fluid in all stages of the disease during acute episode, intercritical period and also in chronic tophaceous gout.

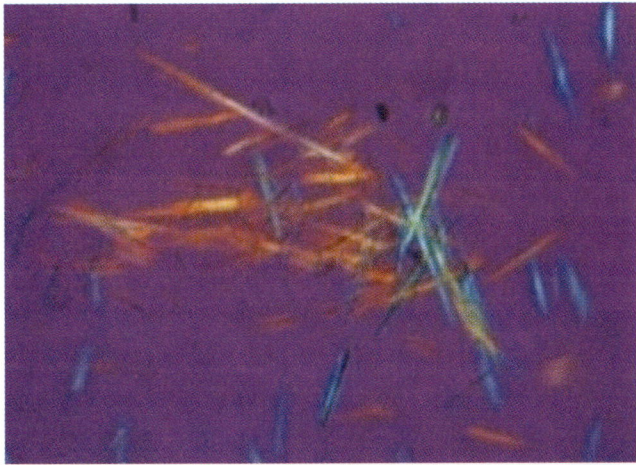

Fig. 29.2: Negatively birefringent crystals of monosodium urate (MSU)

Lesch-Nyhan Syndrome

A 2-year-old male child brought to the hospital with complain of involuntary movements of upper limb and habit of biting of lips and fingers. On examination, baby had multiple marks of biting on fingers and lips (Fig. 29.3). Mother gives the history of orangish discoloration of baby diaper.

Following were the investigation report:
- Serum uric acid: 9 mg/dL

Comment on the diagnosis.

Explanation

LNS (Lesch-Nyhan syndrome) is an **'X-linked recessive'** disorder of purine metabolism which affects male child exclusively. In this disorder, individual demonstrates spasticity, choreoathetosis, elevated uric acid, self-injurious, and aggressive behavior.

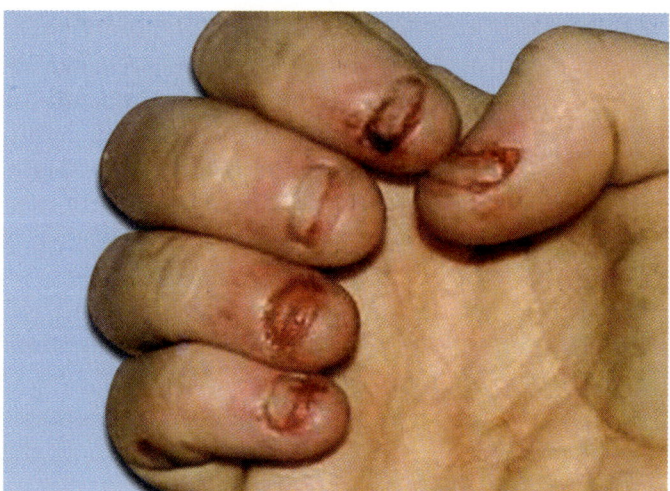

Fig. 29.3: Self-mutilation in a case of Lesch-Nyhan syndrome

This syndrome is associated with deficient activity of the enzyme **hypoxanthine guanine phosphoribosyl transferase (HGPRT)** an enzyme of purine nucleotide salvage pathway. In deficiency of this enzyme, excess hypoxanthine is diverted for degradation and uric acid formation (Fig. 29.4).

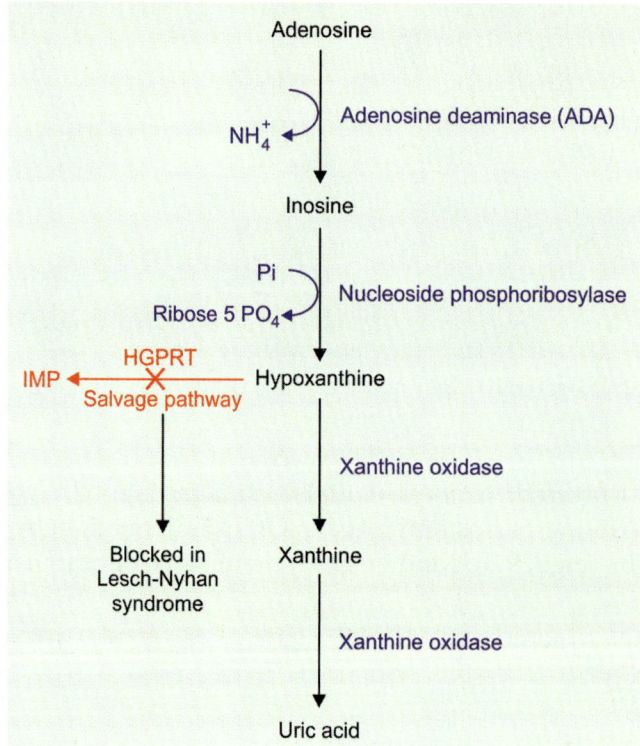

Fig. 29.4: HGPRT enzyme and salvage hypoxanthine to IMP

At birth, most individuals with LNS show normal motor development, but by 6–8 months begin to display signs of progressive generalized spastic paresis and bilateral athetosis.

Notes

CHAPTER

30

Interpretation of Laboratory Result: Arterial Blood Gas (ABG) Analysis

Competency

BI 6.8: Discuss and interpret results of arterial blood gas (ABG) analysis in various disorders.

ACID-BASE DISORDER: A GENERAL OVERVIEW

Normal systemic pH is 7.35 to 7.45. Intracellular and extracellular buffer system as well as organ systems like respiratory and renal systems play important role in maintaining the pH in this range.

$PaCO_2$ (partial pressure of CO_2) is controlled by respiratory system and plasma bicarbonate (HCO_3^-) is controlled by renal system.

Henderson-Hasselbalch equation denotes the inter-relation of $PaCO_2$ (partial pressure of CO_2) and plasma bicarbonate (HCO_3^-) on plasma pH (Fig. 30.1).

$$pH = 6.1 + \frac{\log HCO_3}{PCO_2 \times 0.03001}$$

Fig. 30.1: Henderson-Hasselbalch equation

The compensatory response in the change of plasma bicarbonate (HCO_3^-) in metabolic acidosis is by change in $PaCO_2$ (partial pressure of CO_2) in the same direction as to maintain the ratio of HCO_3 and PCO_2 concentration. Same holds true for change in $PaCO_2$ in respiratory disorder where plasma bicarbonate (HCO_3^-) is moved to same direction as that of $PaCO_2$ as to maintain the ratio of HCO_3 and PCO_2 concentration.

In other words, in a **simple acid-base disorder**, change in plasma bicarbonate (HCO_3^-) and $PaCO_2$ (partial pressure of CO_2) go hand in hand, means when the plasma bicarbonate (HCO_3^-) declines in a case of metabolic acidosis then $PaCO_2$ (partial pressure of CO_2) also declines via hyperventilation as a compensatory response and vice versa. Degree of respiratory compensation in a case of metabolic acidosis is predicted by following equation:

$$PaCO_2 = [HCO_3^-] + 15$$

Thus, in a patient with metabolic acidosis with plasma bicarbonate (HCO_3^-) level of 15 mmol/L, $PaCO_2$ (partial pressure of CO_2) is expected to be 30 mm Hg. Any derangement in the level of $PaCO_2$ from expected value denotes mixed disturbance.

If the change in PaCO₂ and plasma bicarbonate (HCO₃⁻) is in opposite direction, it denotes mixed acid-base disturbance.

Normal serum level of:
- pH: 7.35 to 7.45
- Plasma bicarbonate (HCO₃⁻): 22 to 26 mmol/L
- PaCO₂ (partial pressure of CO₂): 35 to 45 mm Hg
- H₂CO₃: 1.2 mEq/L
- PaO₂ (partial pressure of O₂): 85 to 105 mm Hg
- O₂ saturation: 95 to 100%

Metabolic Acidosis

Key features in ABG analysis in metabolic acidosis are:
- Low pH
- Low plasma bicarbonate (HCO₃⁻)
- Low PaCO₂ due to compensatory hyperventilation (increased tidal volume: Kussmaul respiration)

Metabolic acidosis may be due to:
- Increased endogenous acid production (ketoacidosis, lactic acidosis)
- Loss of plasma bicarbonate (HCO₃⁻) (diarrhea)
- Low excretion of net acid by kidney (in chronic kidney disease)

Metabolic acidosis may be high anion gap or non-anion gap type.

Anion Gap

In the plasma, sum of total anion is equal to sum of total cation. It is not possible to measure all the anions in plasma and anion gap denotes this unmeasured anion which is represented by following formula (Fig. 30.2).

$$AG = [Na^+ + K^+] - [HCO_3 - Cl]$$

Fig. 30.2: Anion gap calculation

Unmeasured anions normally found in plasma are albumin, sulfate, phosphate and organic ions. Normal value of anion gap is 10–12 mmol/L.

Causes of high anion gap metabolic acidosis:
- Ketoacidosis (diabetes, starvation, alcohol)
- Lactic acidosis
- Toxins (ethylene glycol, methanol, salicylate, propylene glycol)
- Renal failure (acute, chronic)

Causes of non-anion gap metabolic acidosis:
- Loss of bicarbonate through intestine (diarrhea, MgSO₄ therapy)
- Renal tubular acidosis (RTA type 1 and type 2)
- Drug induced (NSAIDs, potassium sparing diuretics, trimethoprim)

Metabolic Alkalosis

Key features in ABG analysis in a case of metabolic alkalosis are:
- Elevated pH
- High plasma bicarbonate (HCO_3^-)
- High $PaCO_2$ due to compensatory alveolar hypoventilation

Metabolic alkalosis may be due to:
- Exogenous bicarbonate administration [milk-alkali syndrome]
- Vomiting
- Gastric aspiration
- Diuretics
- Renal arterial stenosis

Respiratory Acidosis

Key features in ABG analysis in a case of respiratory acidosis are:
- Decreased pH
- Increased $PaCO_2$ due to severe respiratory disease, muscle fatigue
- High plasma bicarbonate (HCO_3^-) as a compensatory mechanism

Respiratory acidosis may be due to:
- Sedatives, head trauma, intracranial tumors
- Airway obstruction, asthma, emphysema
- Polio, myasthenia
- Obesity hypoventilation syndrome
- Hypoventilation

Respiratory Alkalosis

Key features in ABG analysis in a case of respiratory alkalosis are:
- Elevated pH
- Low $PaCO_2$
- Low plasma bicarbonate (HCO_3^-)

Respiratory alkalosis may be due to:
- Anxiety
- Pain
- Fever
- Tumor
- Trauma
- High altitudes
- Pulmonary embolism
- Septicemia

LAB REPORT INTERPRETATION: ARTERIAL BLOOD GAS (ABG)
Case Discussion

Case 1: A 70-year-old diabetic male is brought to casualty in a comatose state. His breath had fruity odor and Kussmaul type of breathing was noticed. Following are the biochemical findings:
- Blood sugar: 375 mg/dL
- Urine ketone body: Positive

ABG (arterial blood gas):
- pH: 7.18 (normal = 7.35 to 7.45)
- Plasma bicarbonate (HCO_3^-): 18 mmol/L (normal = 22 to 26 mmol/L)
- $PaCO_2$ (partial pressure of CO_2): 28 mm Hg (normal = 35 to 45 mm Hg)
- H_2CO_3: 1.2 mEq/L (normal = 1.2 mEq/L)
- PaO_2 (partial pressure of O_2): 89 mm Hg (85 to 105 mm Hg)
- O_2 saturation: 95% (normal = 95 to 100%)
- Na^+ = 140 mEq/L (normal = 135–145 mEq/L)
- K^+ = 4.0 mEq/L (normal = 3.5 to 5.5 mEq/L)
- Cl^- = 102 mEq/L (normal = 95 to 105 mEq/L)

Explanation

This patient is in a state of metabolic acidosis (uncompensated) because of diabetic ketoacidosis.

Key features in ABG analysis in metabolic acidosis are:
- Low pH
- Low plasma bicarbonate (HCO_3^-)
- Low $PaCO_2$ due to compensatory hyperventilation (increased tidal volume: Kussmaul respiration)

Anion gap in this case is [140 + 4] – [102 + 18] = 24.
Normal value of anion gap is 10–12 mmol/L.
So, it is a case of high anion gap acidosis.

Case 2: A 45-year-old patient comes in a state of confusion and altered sensorium. She is having copious vomiting for past two days. She is a known patient of duodenal ulcer obstruction (DUO). Following are the ABG reports.

ABG (arterial blood gas):
- pH: 7.7 [normal = 7.35 to 7.45]
- Plasma bicarbonate (HCO_3^-): 38 mmol/L [normal = 22 to 26 mmol/L]
- $PaCO_2$ (partial pressure of CO_2): 52 mm Hg [normal = 35 to 45 mm Hg]
- H_2CO_3: 1.2 mEq/L [normal = 1.2 mEq/L]
- PaO_2 (partial pressure of O_2): 92 mm Hg [85 to 105 mm Hg]
- O_2 saturation: 96% [normal = 95 to 100%]

Interpret above ABG report.

Explanation

Patient is suffering with metabolic alkalosis [uncompensated].
Key features in ABG analysis in metabolic alkalosis are:
- Elevated pH

- High plasma bicarbonate (HCO_3^-)
- High $PaCO_2$ due to compensatory alveolar hypoventilation

Case 3: A 24-year-old male is coming in a comatose state following road traffic accident. He has sustained fracture skull. Following are the ABG reports.

ABG (arterial blood gas):
- pH: 7.20 [normal = 7.35 to 7.45]
- Plasma bicarbonate (HCO_3^-): 34 mmol/L [normal = 22 to 26 mmol/L]
- $PaCO_2$ (partial pressure of CO_2): 85 mm Hg [normal = 35 to 45 mm Hg]
- H_2CO_3: 2.1 mEq/L [normal = 1.2 mEq/L]
- PaO_2 (partial pressure of O_2): 89 mm Hg [85 to 105 mm Hg]
- O_2 saturation: 95% [normal= 95 to 100%]

Interpret the report.

Explanation

Patient is suffering with respiratory acidosis [uncompensated].

Key features of respiratory acidosis in ABG analysis are:
- Decreased pH
- Increased $PaCO_2$
- High plasma bicarbonate (HCO_3^-) as a compensatory mechanism

Case 4: A 17-year-old female came to casualty with hyperventilation. She was anxious and was having carpopedal spasm in fingers. Similar episodes were reported previously for which she was hospitalized and was completely cured. Attendants are not able to comment on diagnosis or management protocol. Following are the ABG reports.

ABG (arterial blood gas):
- pH: 7.6 [normal = 7.35 to 7.45]
- Plasma bicarbonate (HCO_3^-): 20 mmol/L [normal = 22 to 26 mmol/L]
- $PaCO_2$ (partial pressure of CO_2): 22 mm Hg [normal = 35 to 45 mm Hg]
- H_2CO_3: 1.0 mEq/L [normal = 1.2 mEq/L]
- PaO_2 (partial pressure of O_2): 95 mm Hg [85 to 105 mm Hg]
- O_2 saturation: 97% [normal = 95 to 100%]

1. Interpret the result.
2. How do you explain the carpopedal spasm in this condition?

Explanation

This lady is having respiratory alkalosis [uncompensated].
It is due to hyperventilation and CO_2 wash off.

Key features of respiratory alkalosis in ABG analysis are:
- Elevated pH
- Low $PaCO_2$
- Low plasma bicarbonate (HCO_3^-)

Because of raised pH, there is more of the binding of calcium ion to the albumin, this results in lowering of ionized calcium and this results in carpopedal spasm.

Notes

CHAPTER 31

Cerebrospinal Fluid (CSF)

Competency

BI 11.15: Describe and discuss the composition of CSF.

Q1. What is CSF (cerebrospinal fluid)?
Ans. CSF is ultrafiltrate of plasma which is clear and colorless liquid. It surrounds the brain and spinal cord. CSF flows in between arachnoid and pia mater, an area known as subarachnoid space. Total volume of CSF in a normal healthy adult is 150 mL. Per day 500 mL of CSF is synthesized and synthesis results because of selective ultrafiltration of plasma and active secretion by the epithelial membrane.

Q2. What is the function of CSF?
Ans. Three major functions of CSF are:
1. *Physical support and protection*: This is the major function of CSF, whereby it provides a cushion around the brain and spinal cord and dissipates any thrust or shock.
2. *Providing controlled chemical environment* which supplies nutrient to tissues and removes the waste: As this is the ultrafiltrate of plasma which differs in its constituent, but the constituents are maintained within the narrow limit.
3. *Intracerebral and extracerebral transportation*: Hypophyseal hormones are distributed within the brain and hormone from brain is cleared and is send to the cell.

Q3. What are the indications of CSF analysis?
Ans. Following are the indications of CSF analysis:
a. CNS infection
b. Demyelinating disease {subacute sclerosing panencephalitis (SSPE), multiple sclerosis}
c. Hemorrhages in CNS
d. Malignancy

Q4. How the CSF sample is collected for analysis?
Ans. CSF can be collected by lumbar puncture done under strict aseptic precaution. Interspace of vertebrae L3–L4 or lower.

20 mL of CSF can be collected safely though this much amount is not required for analysis. Sample is divided in three aliquots for:
a. Chemistry and serology,

b. Microbiology, and
   c. Hematology.

Q5. What is the normal appearance of CSF? How the appearance of CSF is important in hinting the diagnosis?

Ans. Normally, CSF is clear, colorless liquid, free of blood, free of clot. In CNS infection (which may be bacterial/viral/fungal infection), the appearance of CSF is cloudy. If there is blood in CSF which may be because of traumatic puncture or subarachnoid hemorrhage, it shows yellow-brown-red discoloration.

Q6. In CSF analysis, what are all serological parameters being done?

Ans. Following are the serological parameters which are analyzed in CSF:

a. Glucose
b. Lactate
c. Protein (total and specific)
d. Glutamine

a. *Glucose*: Glucose is carried by specific carriers in the CSF fluid. Normally, the level of CSF glucose is 2/3rd of plasma glucose. It ranges between 40 and 85 mg/dL based on plasma glucose. Simultaneous blood glucose assessment is important to have correct interpretation.

   Increased glucose in CSF denotes hyperglycemia and clinically not very significant.

   Decreased glucose in CSF (hypoglycorrhachia) may be due to:
   a. Active metabolism of glucose by cell or microorganism (bacterial, fungal, amebic)
   b. Disorder of carrier-mediated transport [in tuberculosis (TB) and in sarcoidosis]
   c. Consumption by the CNS due to increased metabolism (brain tumor, diffuse meningeal malignancy)

b. *Lactate*: Consumption of glucose by cell or organism is associated with increased lactate level. Increased lactate with decreased level of glucose is indicative of bacterial meningitis.

c. *Protein*: Total protein in the CSF is 0.5% or 1/100 to that of the plasma.

   Normal CSF protein concentration is 15 to 45 mg/dL.

   80% of CSF protein originates from ultrafiltrate of plasma and remaining 20% is originated due to intrathecal synthesis.

   Increase of CSF protein is seen in following conditions:
   - In bacterial meningitis, it exceeds 100 mg/dL.
   - In viral meningitis, it is raised to 20–80 mg/dL.
   - In mechanical obstruction by spinal tumor, it raises to the extent of 100 to 2000 mg/dL.
   - In addition to above conditions, TB meningitis, hemorrhages, multiple sclerosis, etc. result in increased level of protein in the CSF.

   Decrease of CSF protein is seen in following conditions:
   - Increased leakage of CSF from tear of dura mater
   - Decreased dialysis from plasma
   - Excess CSF removal

d. *Glutamine*: It is elevated in hepatic encephalopathy when more of the glutamine formation is seen in brain. Plasma ammonia is though the better indicator of hepatic encephalopathy compared to CSF glutamine level.

   CSF parameters in various diseases is represented in Table 31.1.

Table 31.1: CSF parameters in various diseases

Parameters	Normal CSF	Bacterial meningitis	Viral meningitis	TB meningitis
Glucose (mg/dL)	40–85	<40 (may be zero)	Normal	<50
Protein (mg/dL)	15–45	>100	20–80	100–200
WBC (per µL)	<5	>1000	25–500	25–500

Q7. What are the precautions which need to be taken while analyzing CSF?

Ans. Following precautions may be taken while analyzing the CSF:

a. Blood specimen should be obtained 3 to 4 hours before collecting the CSF sample as to have comparative analysis of various analyte and proper interpretation.
b. CSF sample should be inspected for its physical appearance before the centrifugation.
c. Immediate analysis of CSF is done specially for estimation of glucose content as otherwise the consumption of glucose by bacteria may alter the value of glucose in CSF.

Notes

Notes

Section VI

Vitamin and Mineral Deficiencies and Their Clinical Manifestation (Chart Discussion/Spotter)

32. Water-Soluble Vitamins
33. Fat-Soluble Vitamins
34. Minerals and Clinical Manifestation of Their Plasma Level Derangements

Competencies

DR 17.1: Enumerate and identify the cutaneous findings in vitamin A deficiency.
DR 17.2: Enumerate and describe the various skin changes in vitamin B complex deficiency.
DR 17.3: Enumerate and describe the various changes in vitamin C deficiency.
DR 17.4: Enumerate and describe the various changes in zinc deficiency.
PE 12.3: Identify the clinical features of dietary deficiency/excess of vitamin A.
PE 12.8: Identify the clinical features of dietary deficiency of vitamin D.
PE 12.17: Identify the clinical features of vitamin B complex deficiency.
PE 12.21: Identify the clinical features of vitamin C deficiency.
PE 13.3: Identify the clinical features of dietary deficiency of iron and make a diagnosis.
PE 13.9: Identify the clinical features of iodine deficiency disorders.

CHAPTER

32

Water-Soluble Vitamins

Vitamin C: Scurvy

A 42-year-old male presented with history of bleeding gums and petechial hemorrhages on skin. His diet consisted of mainly carbohydrates which lacked fresh fruits and vegetables. On examination, gums are swollen and bleeding was visible (Fig. 32.1).

Blood vitamin C levels were 0.11 mg/dL (normal levels: 0.20 to 2.00 mg/dL).

Vitamin C supplements were administered with dramatic improvement in the symptoms.
1. **What is the most probable diagnosis in this case?**
2. **What is the reason of bleeding gum in this person?**
3. **Explain the role of vitamin C in collagen synthesis?**
4. **Write dietary sources rich in vitamin C?**

Explanation

1. This patient is suffering with scurvy, a condition which arises due to deficiency of vitamin C.
2 and 3. Vitamin C is necessary for synthesis of collagen which is important for blood vessel wall formation. Vitamin C is needed for action of **prolyl hydroxylase and lysyl hydroxylase** enzymes

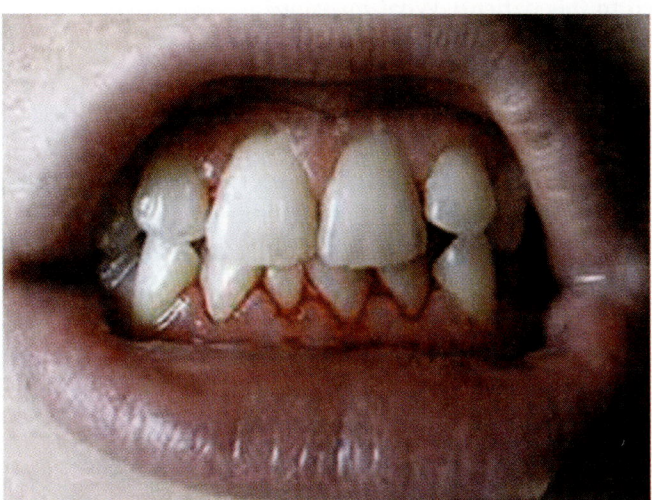

Fig. 32.1: Scurvy bleeding gum

which are needed for conversion of proline and lysine to hydroxyproline and hydroxylysine, respectively.

This conversion of amino acid is important to stabilize the structure of collagen. In deficiency of vitamin C, structure of collagen is not stable and that results in weakening of blood vessel wall and fragility which is manifested in gums and also on skin as ecchymosis.

4. Most abundant source of vitamin C is Indian gooseberry (Amla) followed by guava and lime (Fig. 32.2).

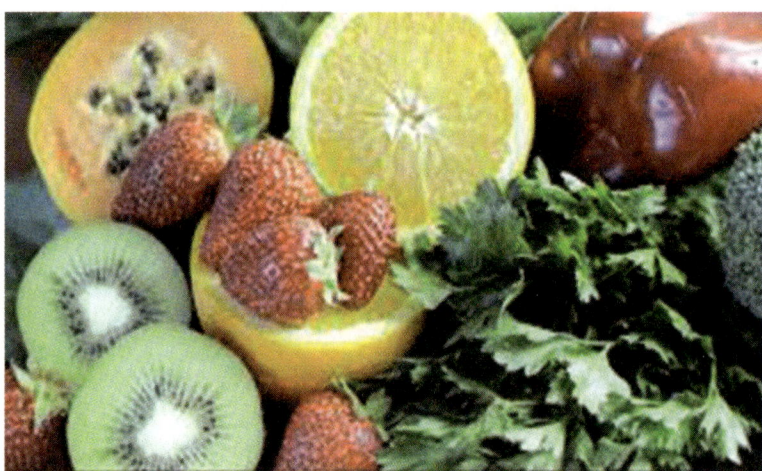

Fig. 32.2: Food rich in vitamin C

Wernicke-Korsakoff Psychosis: Vitamin B_1

A 56-year-old male belonging to poor socioeconomic strata presents with the history of forgetfulness, muscle weakness, poor appetite, and tremors in hand and nystagmus (involuntary eye movements). He is a known alcoholic for past 20 years. On examination, he was found to have unsteady gate and fine tremors. He was found to have mental confusion too.

1. What is the probable diagnosis in above case?
2. What nutrient deficiency may be suspected in above case?
3. How will you approach to this patient? What investigation would you require to confirm the diagnosis and what will be the treatment plan?

Explanation

1. and 2. This seems to be a case of **"Wernicke-Korsakoff psychosis"** which is due to moderately severe deficiency of vitamin B_1 (thiamine). This is seen in chronic alcoholic and is due to poor diet intake and also due to impaired absorption of nutrients from gastrointestinal tract.

Mild deficiency of vitamin presents with loss of appetite, fatigue, irritability, peripheral neuropathy and is seen in elderly with poor diet intake.

Moderately severe deficiency is reflected in symptoms of 'Wernicke-Korsakoff psychosis' described above. **Wernicke disease** is characterized by **clinical triad of global confusion, ophthalmoplegia, and ataxia.** This classic triad is seen only in 1/3rd of patients presenting clinically (Fig. 32.3).

Korsakoff psychosis is the amnestic state where patient shows impairment of recent memory, though the past memory remains intact. Confabulation is an important characteristic where patient fills the memory gap by falsification which he believes to be true.

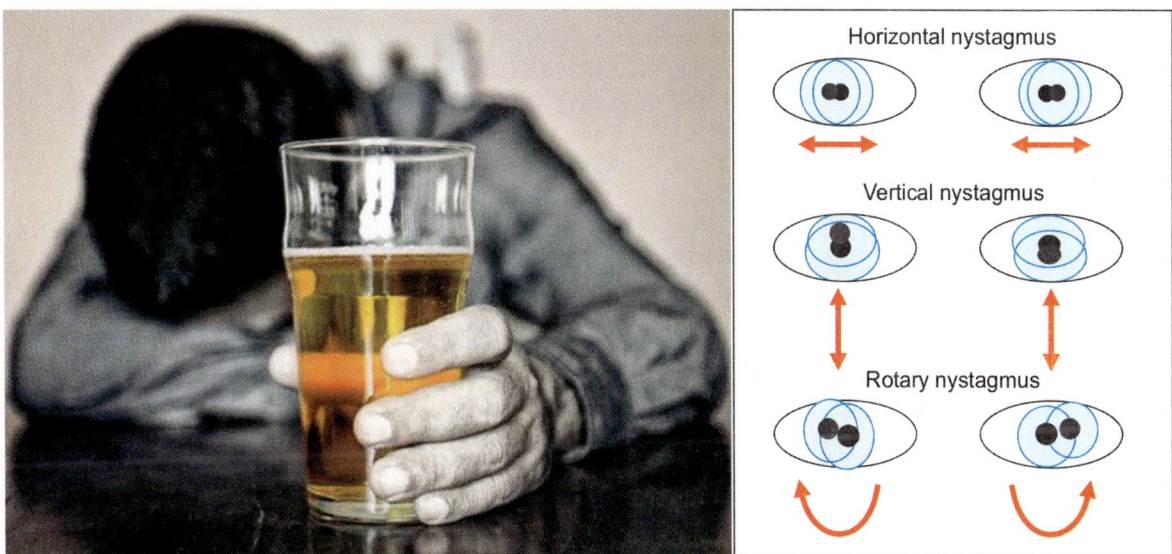

Fig. 32.3: Alcoholic person and nystagmus in eye

There is irreversible damage at medial thalamic nucleic and mammillary bodies in the brain. MRI shows mammillary body atrophy in chronic phase.

Severe deficiency of vitamin B_1 is rare but manifests in form of 'beriberi' which is described in the next case.

3. Vitamin B_1 level can be estimated in plasma. **RBC transketolase activity** may be assessed to find out vitamin B_1 deficiency. Patient may be given vitamin B_1 supplementation with other supportive therapy.

Wet Beriberi: Vitamin B_1

A 5-year-old male child of a labour presents with lethargy, poor appetite, irritability and pitting **pedal edema**. His family is mainly relying on carbohydrate diet consisting of polished rice (Figs 32.4 and 32.5).

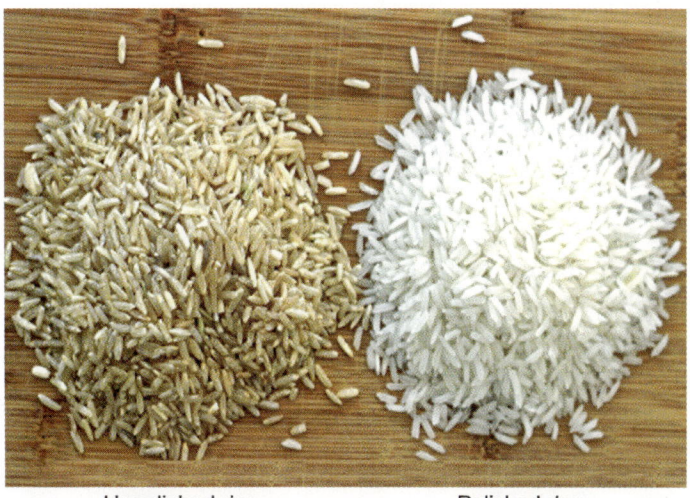

Fig. 32.4: Polished and unpolished rice

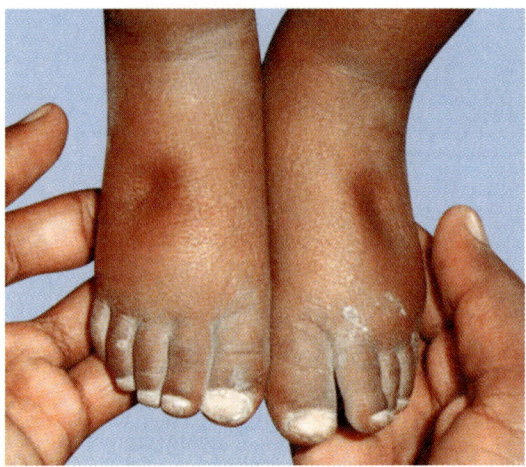

Fig. 32.5: Pitting pedal edema

Q. What is the probable diagnosis in this case? What may the possible vitamin deficiency in this child? How the consumption of polished rice is related to the symptoms in this baby?

Explanation

This baby seems to have **beriberi**, a disease which is seen in severe case of **vitamin B$_1$ (thiamine) deficiency**. Beriberi may be:

a. **Dry beriberi**, characterized by neuromuscular symptoms, muscular atrophy and emaciation.
b. **Wet beriberi**, characterized by symptoms of dry beriberi but in addition will have pedal edema.

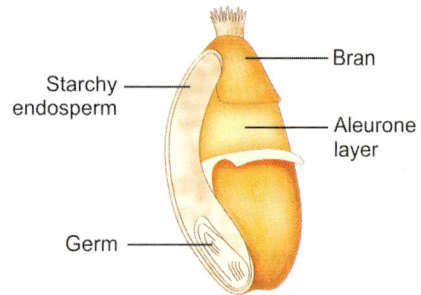

Fig. 32.6: Aleurone layer of cereal

Vitamin B$_1$ is found in outer **aleurone layer of cereals**. On polishing, the rice's outer layer is removed and along with that even vitamin B$_1$ is lost (Fig. 32.6).

Consumption of polished rice results in vitamin B$_1$ deficiency, hence unpolished rice is healthier to consume.

Ariboflavinosis: Vitamin B$_2$ Deficiency

A 12-year-old boy presenting with the history of repeated attack of ulceration at the corner of mouth and swollen painful tongue. He is a vegetarian.

On examination, his lips were dry and there was ulceration at the corner of mouth which was making it difficult for him to open the mouth completely. Tongue was red and swollen. Examination of eye showed **circumcorneal vascularization** (Fig. 32.7).

1. What is the vitamin deficiency associated with these symptoms?
2. What is the dietary source of this vitamin?
3. What is the RDA of this vitamin?

Explanation

Vitamin B$_2$ (riboflavin) deficiency is associated with above manifestation. Liver, yeast, egg, milk, fish, and cereals are good sources of vitamin B$_2$.

RDA of vitamin B$_2$ is 1.5 mg/dL.

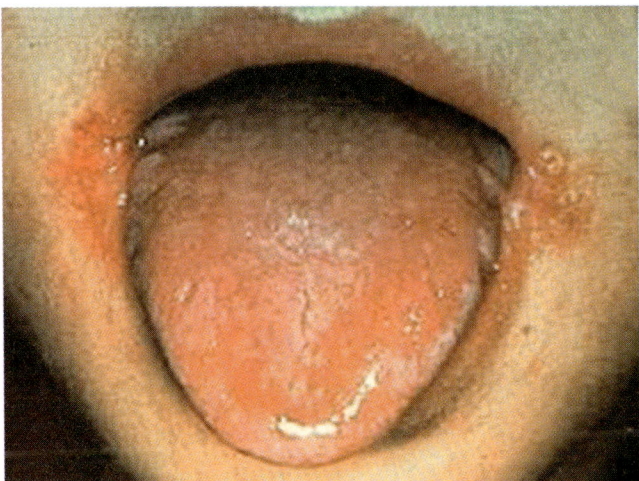

Fig. 32.7: Swollen tongue and cracks at corner of mouth (ariboflavinosis)

B_2 deficiency is manifested in the form for glossitis, angular stomatitis, dry scaly lips, circumcorneal vascularization, and bulbar conjunctiva proliferation.

Pellagra: Vitamin B_3 Deficiency

A 35-year-old poor labour on irregular diet is presenting with the history of frequent diarrhea and dry scaly lesions around the neck for past 6 months. On examination, he was found to have characteristic lesions around the neck and dorsum of hand (Fig. 32.8).

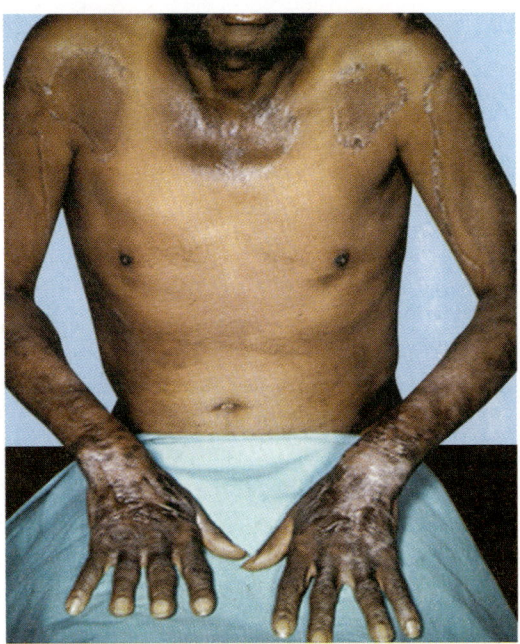

Fig. 32.8: Characteristic dermatitis (Casal necklace and gloved hand) in a typical case of pellagra

1. Name the vitamin deficiency which may be associated with above symptoms.
2. What is the name given to this characteristic lesion observed around the neck of the individual?
3. What is the coenzyme form of the vitamin related in this case?

Explanation

This patient is suffering with pellagra. A disease characterized by **3Ds: Diarrhea, dermatitis and dementia**. In extreme case, patient may die also.

Skin shows characteristic lesion around neck named as **Casal necklace deformity** and dry scaly lesions on hand known as **gloved hand deformity (Fig. 32.9)**.

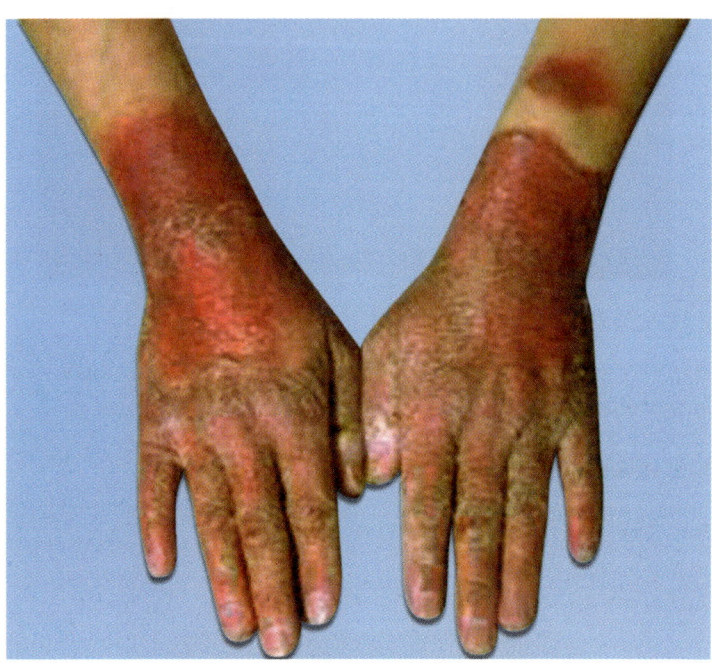

Fig. 32.9: Gloved hand deformity

Vitamin B_6 Deficiency

A 34-year-old engineer coming with complain of tingling and numbness in peripheries. His scalp is dry and scaly. He is a patient of pulmonary tuberculosis on treatment with ATT (antitubercular treatment) for past 3 months.

1. What vitamin deficiency will you suspect in this patient? Mention certain biochemical roles of this vitamin.
2. What is the RDA of concerned vitamin and what is the therapeutic dose of this vitamin in this case?
3. What metabolite can be assessed in urine to find out the deficiency of vitamin B_6 in this individual?

Explanation

This patient is having symptoms of vitamin B_6 (pyridoxine). Isoniazid is an antitubercular drug which is associated with vitamin B_6 deficiency.

Vitamin B_6 is needed as coenzyme form for transamination, decarboxylation, glycogen metabolism (glycogen synthase and glycogen phosphorylase), heme synthesis (ALA synthase), metabolism of sulfur-containing amino acid (cystathionine beta-synthase and cystathionase).

RDA for vitamin B_6 is 1.5 mg/dL. But for treatment in this case, higher dose is given (50–100 mg/dL/day).

Patients with vitamin B_6 deficiency excrete xanthurenic acid in the urine. Xanthurenic acid is the metabolite synthesized by kynurenine in alternate pathway of tryptophan metabolism when the normal route is impaired due to lack of activity of kynureninase enzyme.

Biotin (Vitamin B_7) Deficiency

A 21-year-old athlete is coming with the complain of loss of hair, red scaly rash around the mouth, nose, and eyes and tingling sensation on extremities. He gives the history of consumption of 4 to 5 raw eggs in a day for past 6 months as he has to participate in an athletic event in near future.

Q. What is vitamin deficiency suspected in this case?

Explanation

- Biotin (vitamin B_7) deficiency is suspected in this case.
- Source of biotin is egg yolk, liver, cereals, spinach, mushrooms and rice.
- Biotin deficiency presents with periorificial dermatitis, alopecia.
- Skin lesion resembles zinc deficiency lesions.
- Five carboxylases: Pyruvate carboxylase (gluconeogenesis), beta-methylcrotonyl-CoA carboxylase and propionyl-CoA carboxylase (amino acid metabolism) and acetyl-CoA carboxylase 1 and 2 (fatty acid synthesis) need biotin.
- Treatment with oral biotin is beneficial (5 mg/day).
- Biotinidase deficiency is an autosomal recessive disorder which results in deficiency of biotin as the biotin is not released from dietary protein.

Vitamin B_{12} Deficiency

A 24-year-old female who is strict vegetarian presents with the history of easy tiredness and weakness. On examination, she is pale and peripheral smear shows megaloblastic anemia (Fig. 32.10).

1. Which vitamin deficiency may be suspected in above case?
2. What enzymes need vitamin B_{12} as cofactor?

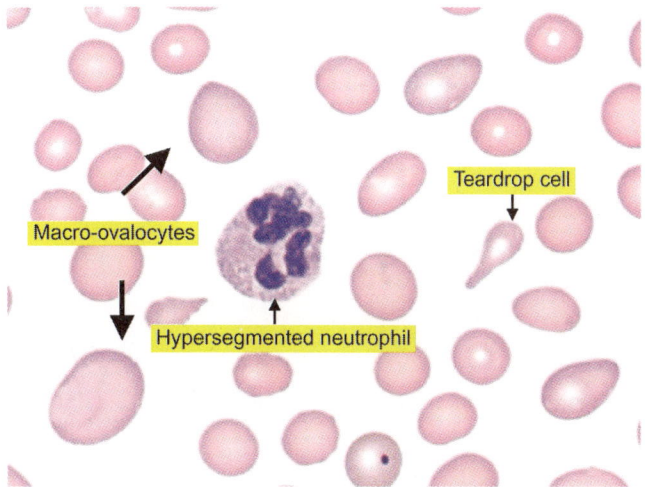

Fig. 32.10: Megaloblastic anemia

Explanation

1. Deficiency of vitamin B_{12} is suspected in this case as the patient is purely vegetarian and vitamin B_{12} is obtained only from foods of animal origin like meat, fish and dairy products.
2. Vitamin B_{12} is cobalt-containing vitamin needed for two important enzymes:
    - Methylmalonyl-CoA mutase (vitamin B_{12} needed is **2-deoxyadenosyl (ado) cobalamin**
    - Methionine synthase (vitamin B_{12} needed in **methylcobalamin** form)

Notes

CHAPTER

33

Fat-Soluble Vitamins

VITAMIN A

Vitamin A Deficiency

A 4-year-old child presents with history of decreased vision after sunset. Mother gives the history of repeated upper respiratory infection in the child. On examination, he was found to have follicular hyperkeratosis on the back of the arm (Fig. 33.1).

Eye examination revealed dry eye (xerophthalmia) and white patches on sclera (Fig. 33.2).

1. **What micronutrient deficiency may be the reason of such presentation in this child? What may be the reason of follicular hyperkeratosis in this child?**
2. **What is the name given to the eye manifestation? What dietary advice to be given for this child?**

Explanation

This child is suffering with vitamin A deficiency. People deficient in this vitamin are prone for repeated infection as the vitamin A is responsible for downregulation of keratin synthesis.

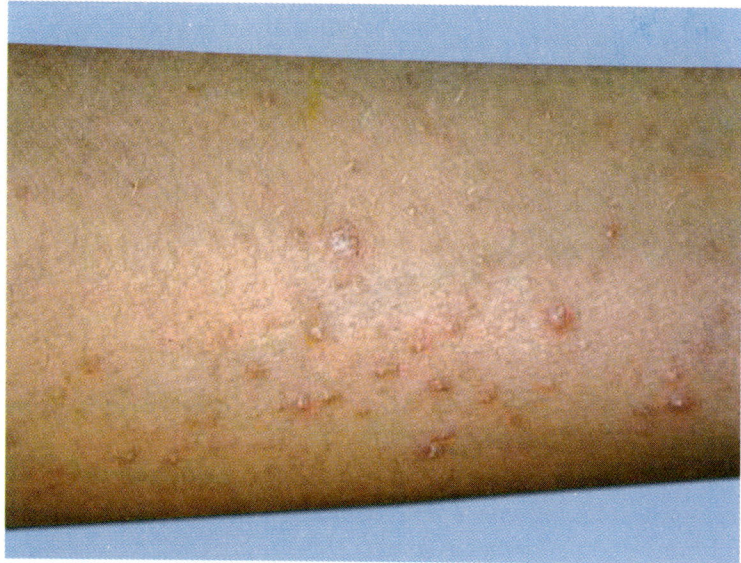

Fig. 33.1: Follicular hyperkeratosis

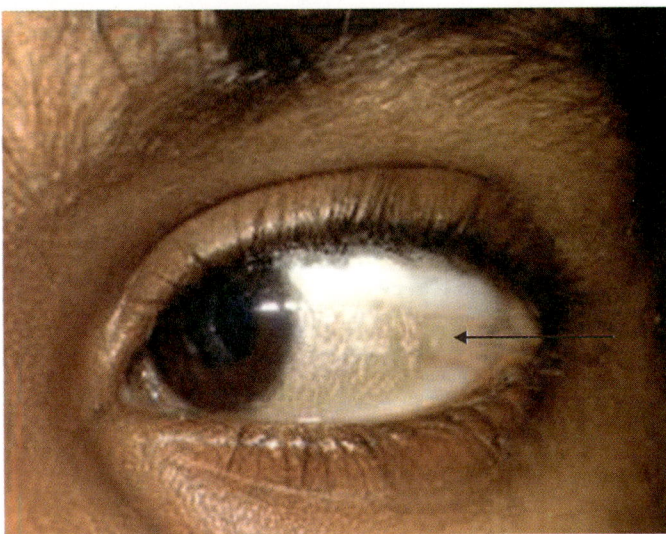

Fig. 33.2: Bitot's spot

In deficiency of vitamin A, there is excessive keratinization of skin and mucous membrane. In skin, it shows up as follicular hyperkeratosis and in mucous membrane of respiratory, gastrointestinal and genitourinary tracts such keratinization favour colonization of microorganism and infection.

In eye, the specific name given to these white patches are **Bitot's spot** which are patches of keratinized epithelium on the sclera (Fig. 33.2).

Vitamin A deficiency poses increased risk of death from diarrhea, dysentery, malaria or respiratory disease.

Yellow and green vegetables have rich amount of vitamin A. For example, mango, banana, carrot, tomato, green leafy vegetable, and pumpkin are good sources of vitamin A (Fig. 33.3).

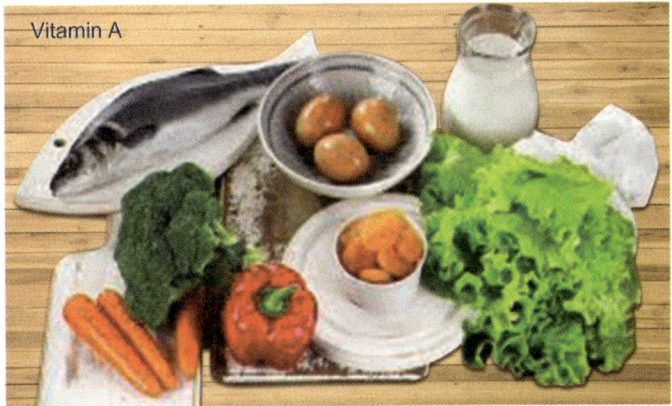

Fig. 33.3: Vitamin A rich fruit

VITAMIN D

Osteomalacia

A 55-year-old postmenopausal female came with complain of backache. On examination, kyphosis was seen. X-ray long bones showed porous matrix. She reported two episodes of fracture small bones of foot in last 3 years.

1. What may be the probable diagnosis in this case?
2. What other investigations you will advise in this case?
3. Which age group is affected by above disease and why?

Explanation

This woman is having **osteomalacia** as obvious in X-ray finding where loss of osteoid matrix is seen.

Hypocalcemia and hypophosphatemia which accompany vitamin D deficiency results in impaired mineralization of bone matrix protein. Hypomineralized matrix results in bowing of weight-bearing extremities and skeletal fractures. Severe vitamin deficiency also causes proximal myopathy in both children and adults (Fig. 33.4).

Pseudo-fractures or looser zones are specific finding in osteomalacia seen in scapula, pelvis and femoral neck.

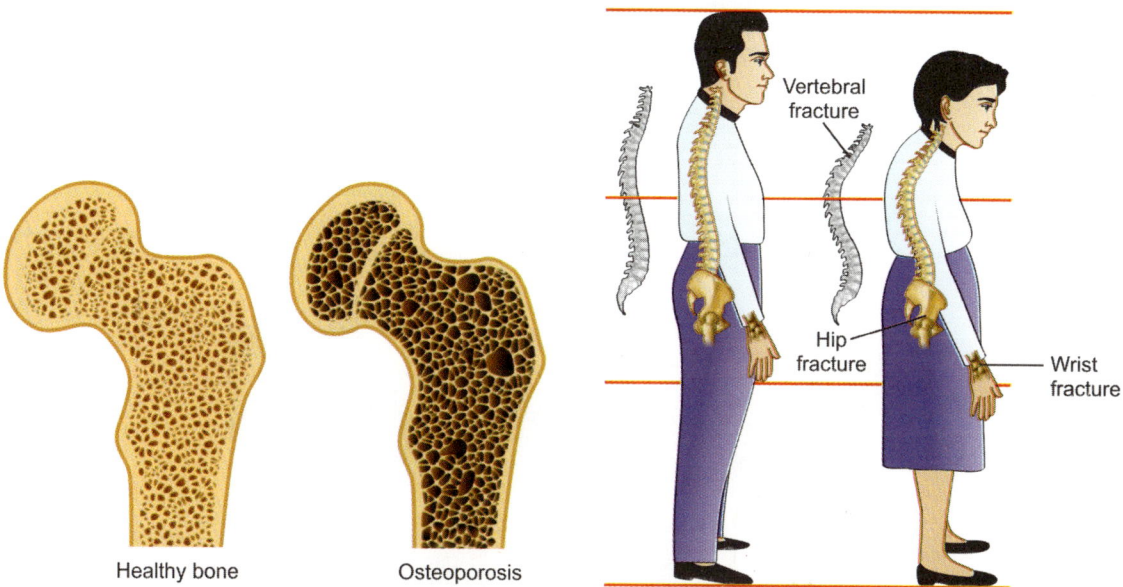

Fig. 33.4: Porous bone in osteoporosis and kyphosis

Rickets

A 5-year-old baby belonging to low socioeconomic strata presented to pediatric OPD with bone deformity of weight-bearing bones and widening of wrist (Fig. 33.5). Chest was prominent on examination.
1. Identify the given disorder.
2. Which micronutrient deficiency will lead to this disorder?
3. Write two biochemical parameters which gets altered in this disorder.
4. Which age group gets affected by this disorder?

Explanation

This child is suffering with deficiency of vitamin D, which results in a disease known as rickets. This condition is very common in India specially in children belonging to poor socioeconomic strata. **Rickets** is characterized by soft and pliable bone which is due to deficient mineralization

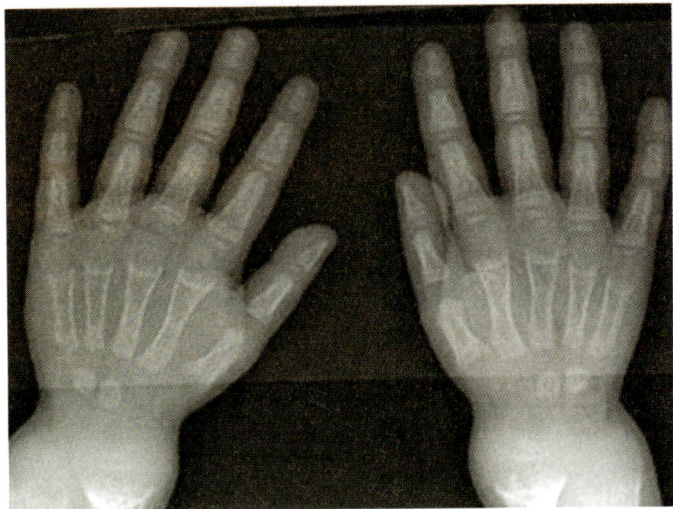

Fig. 33.5: Wrist widening in a child with rickets

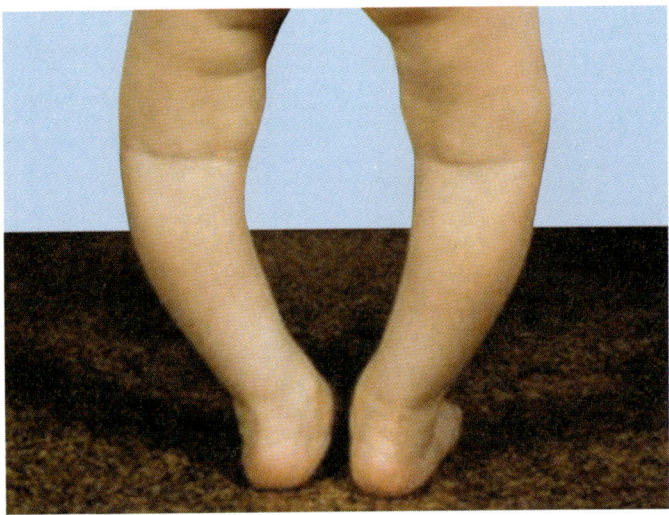

Fig. 33.6: Bow leg in rickets

of the bone. Osteoid matrix and cartilages are formed normally. In children, before the fusion of epiphyseal plate, deficiency of vitamin D results in expansion **(widening) of growth plate** in long bones **(bowed legs)** as well as in **costochondral junction (rachitic rosary)**. Young child of 4 to 6 years mainly suffers with this disease (Figs 33.5 and 33.6).

Level of vitamin D in the plasma can be assessed to know the status of vitamin D in body, and also calcium and phosphorus can be evaluated.

Vitamin D is given in therapeutic doses, along with physiotherapy will be advised.

Vitamin D Toxicity

A 6-year-old child comes with the history of severe headache, vomiting bulging fontanelle. History revealed that the child was treated by a quack for growth retardation, who prescribed him vitamin D injections over a period of more than a year.

X-ray showed metastatic calcification of calf muscle and renal tract stones.

Q. What is the toxic dose of vitamin D? What will be the status of bone mineralization in this toxicity?

Explanation

Upper tolerable limit for vitamin D toxicity is 4000 IU/day in adults and in children, it is 2000 IU/day.

Bone will be demineralized just like seen in rickets, but this time it is due to excess reabsorption of calcium from the bone rather than deficiency of mineralization of the bone.

High plasma level of 1,25 (OH)$_2$ vitamin D and calcium level are important findings in vitamin D toxicity.

Notes

CHAPTER 34

Minerals and Clinical Manifestation of Their Plasma Level Derangements

Iron Deficiency Anemia

A 10-year-old boy came to the OPD with complain of loss of appetite, early fatigue and lethargy. Mother complained that boy is tired very soon while playing and suffer from headache frequently. On examination, nails were flat and pallor was seen. Peripheral smear showed hypochromic, microcytic picture (Figs 34.1 and 34.2).

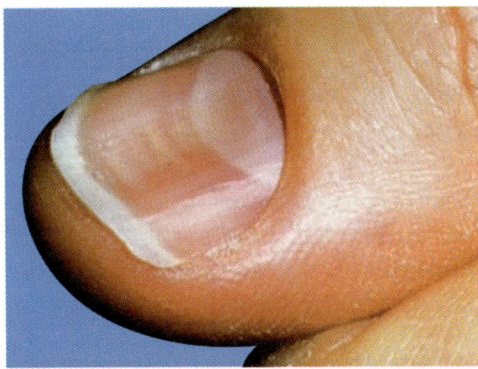

Fig. 34.1: Flat nail in a case of iron deficiency anemia

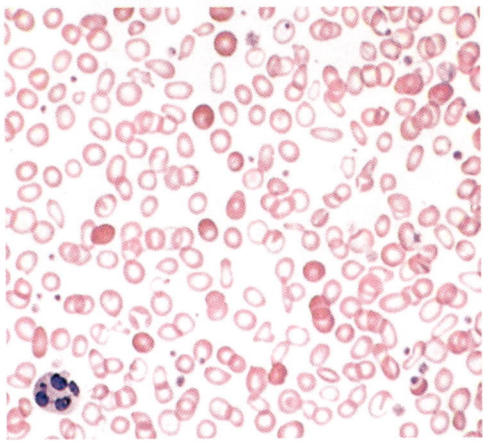

Fig. 34.2: Hypochromic microcytic anemia seen in peripheral smear under microscopic examination

1. What may be the probable diagnosis?
2. Which micronutrient deficiency is related with this disorder?
3. What are the important causes which will lead to this disorder in Indian scenario?

Explanation

This child is suffering with iron deficiency anemia which is characterized by hypochromic microcytic picture of peripheral smear. Lack of iron impairs heme synthesis resulting in hypochromic microcytic picture. Early tiredness is due to inability of RBC to supply sufficient oxygen to tissues (Fig. 34.3).

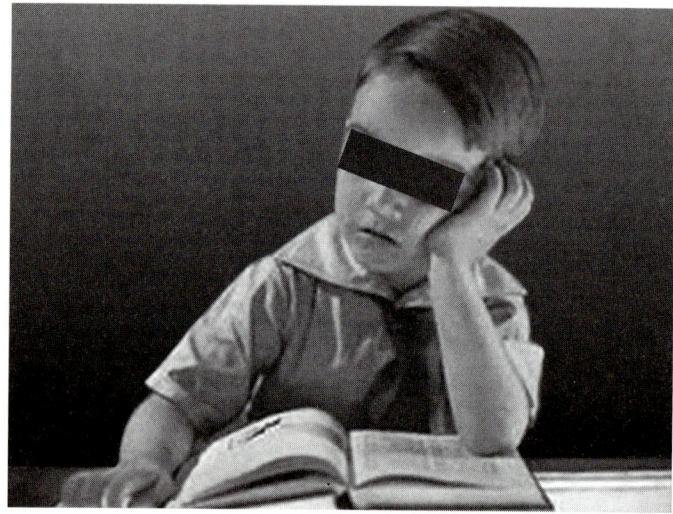

Fig. 34.3: Fatigued child in iron deficiency anemia

Main cause of iron deficiency in Indian scenario is dietary deficiency of iron, superimposed by high phytate content in Indian diet which impair absorption of iron by making insoluble complex with iron. In addition, worm infestation is a major cause of iron deficiency in Indian population. Diet having rich amount of iron are jaggery, black gram, pulses, meat, etc. (Fig. 34.4).

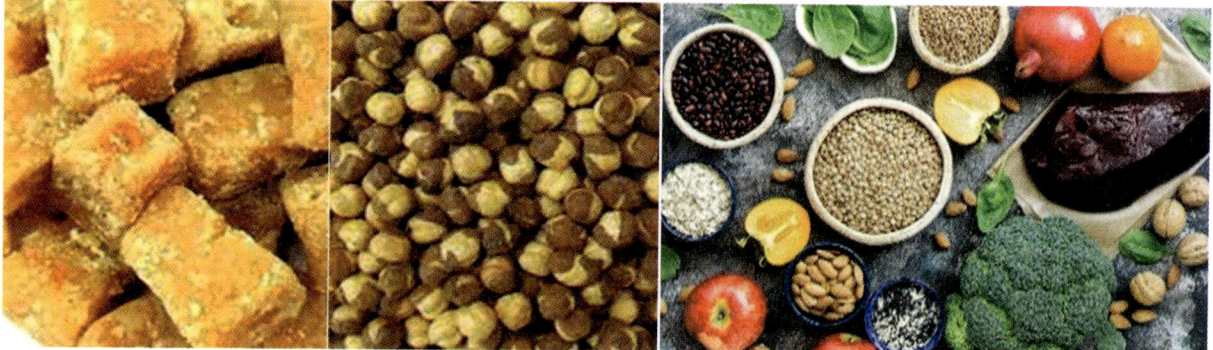

Fig. 34.4: Food items having rich content of iron

Hypocalcemia

A 28-year-old male complain of frequent nocturnal muscle cramps. On physical examination, he showed facial twitching on stroking the cheek. While taking the BP, he developed spasm in fingers as shown in Fig. 34.5.

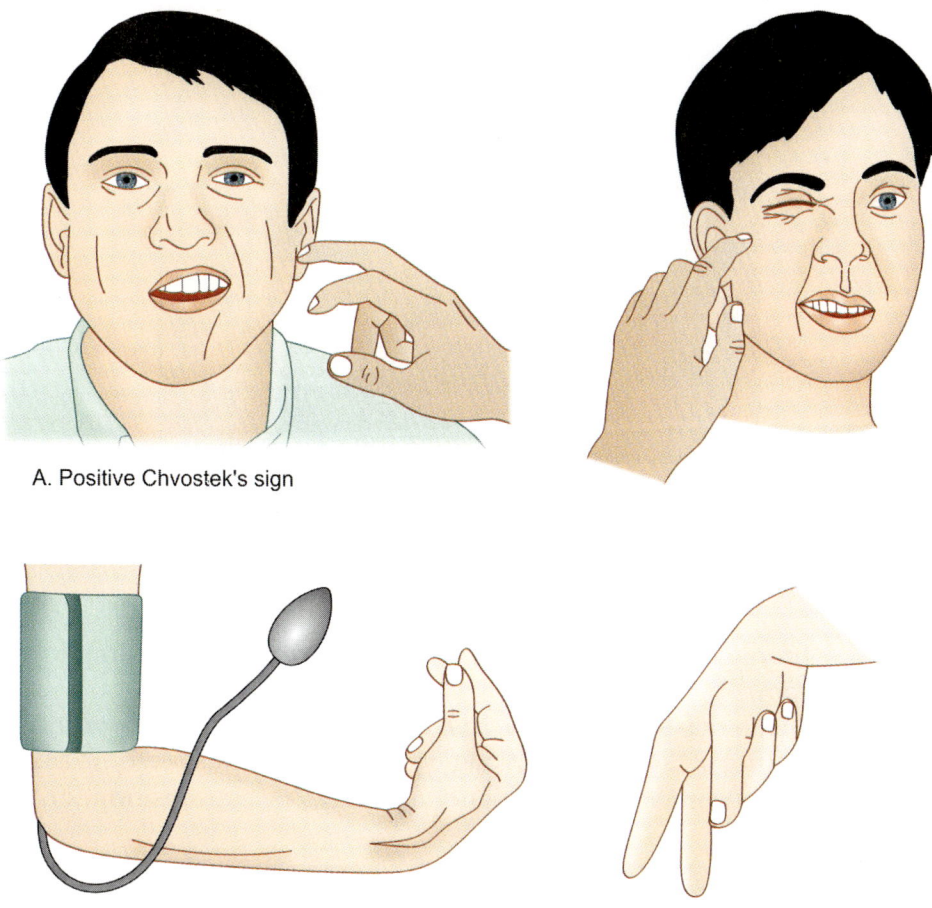

Fig. 34.5: Chvostek's sign and Trousseau's sign

1. Taking into consideration the above illustrated sign and symptoms, what may be the probable clinical diagnosis?
2. Name the above two signs which the patient is showing on examination.
3. Which micronutrient deficiency is related with this disorder?

Explanation
- The presentation in above case is seen typically in hypocalcemia.
- The facial twitching on gently stroking the side of face is known as **Chvostek sign**.
- Adduction of thumb with simultaneous flexion of metacarpophalangeal joints along with extension of interphalangeal joints and flexion of wrist on inflating the BP 20 mm Hg above the systolic pressure for at least 3 minutes is known as **Trousseau's sign**.
- These signs are manifested when the ionized calcium level is less than 4.7 mg/dL. (Normal ionized calcium level is 4.9 mg/dL.)

Fluorosis
An 8-year-old boy presents with bowing of leg and short stature. Many individuals are having similar manifestation in his village. His teeth show mottling and rough ridge (Fig. 34.6).

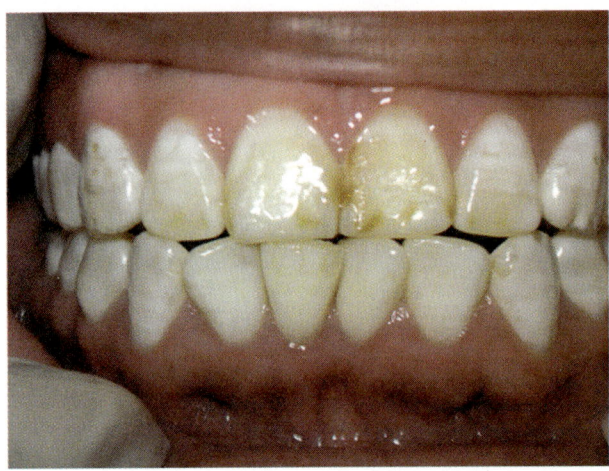

Fig. 34.6: Mottling of teeth in fluorosis

Q. Above manifestation is related with which micronutrient's altered metabolism?

Explanation

This child may be suffering with **fluorosis** which is due to excessive consumption of fluorine in drinking water (>5 ppm).

Daily requirement of fluoride is 1–2 mg, which is easily met with 0.5 to 0.9 ppm level of fluorine in drinking water. Main source of fluoride is drinking water. Sea food and cheese are also good sources.

Fluoride is two-edged sword, and its deficiency as well as excess consumption is related with disease.

Fluoride is needed to strengthen the bone and teeth. Fluorine makes the teeth resistant to cavities, and it strengthens the bone and makes it resistant to osteoporosis. Deficiency (<0.5 ppm fluoride in water) is associated with **dental caries** and **osteoporosis**.

Excess consumption (>5 ppm fluoride in water) is associated with **dental fluorosis** which is characterized by mottled (spotting), discolored teeth with pitting as presented in above case. If the consumption of fluorine is very high for chronic duration (>20 ppm), **skeletal fluorosis** results which is characterized by deformity in bones (Fig. 34.7).

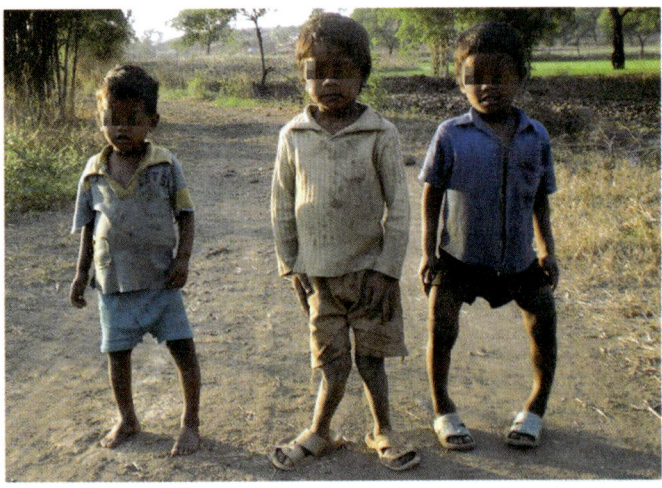

Fig. 34.7: Genu valgum deformity in skeletal fluorosis

Wilson's Disease

A 17-year-old male is admitted to medicine department with history of bizzare behavior, episodes of crying. On examination, he had tremors in hand, incoordinated limb movements, dysarthria and dysphagia was observed. On examination, his eyes showed golden brown ring around corneal rim.

Following were biochemical findings:
- Serum ceruloplasmin: 12 mg/dL (Normal level is 18–35 mg/dL.)
- Copper content in liver (biopsy): 300 µg/g of tissue (Normal level is 20–50 µg/g.)
- Urinary copper (24 hr collection): 270 µg (Normal is 20–50 µg.)

1. Identify the given disorder.
2. Which micronutrient's altered metabolism is related to this kind of manifestation?

Explanation

This patient is suffering with **Wilson's disease** which is autosomal recessive disorder, caused by **mutation of *ATP 7B gene*** which encodes membranous copper transporting ATPase.

The defect in biliary secretion of copper results in excess copper accumulation in liver and toxicity of liver. Level of ceruloplasmin in serum is low due to lack of incorporation of copper to apoceruloplasmin. As the disease advances, free copper in plasma increases which is deposited in brain and eye resulting in neurological and psychiatric disorder, and **Kayser-Fleischer ring** around the cornea. KF ring is visible by naked eye and slit-lamp examination may be needed to confirm the ring (Fig. 34.8).

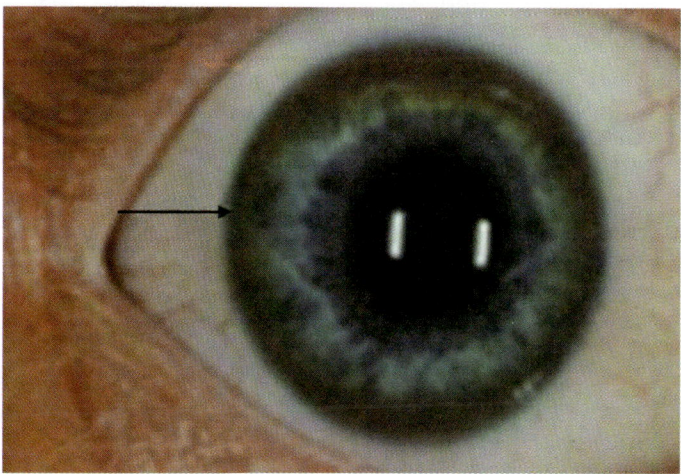

Fig. 34.8: Kayser-Fleischer ring around the cornea due to deposition of Cu in Descemet membrane

Zinc is main line of treatment which not only block the intestinal absorption of copper, it also stimulates the synthesis of metallothionine in the liver which binds the copper in non-toxic form and reduces its toxicity. Penicillamine was used earlier as copper chelator but presently **trientine** is preferred over penicillamine because of its lesser toxicity.

Iron Deficiency Anemia

Case 1: A 24-year-old woman presents with complain of excessive tiredness, poor appetite, inability to do routine work. She gives the history of menorrhagia for past 6 months. On examination, she looks pale, eyes are shrunken and nails are brittle (Fig. 34.9).

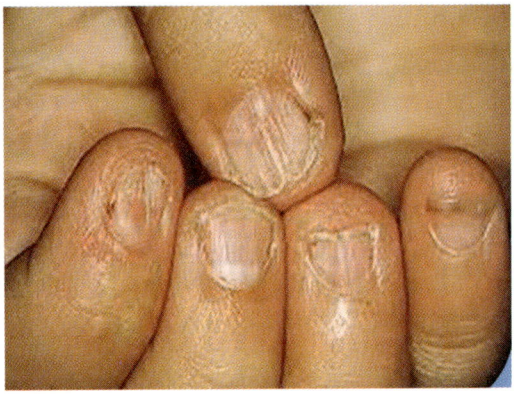

Fig. 34.9: Brittle nail

Laboratory findings are:
- Hemoglobin: 6.5 g/dL [normal 12–14 g/dL]
- Serum iron: 46 ng/dL [normal 50–150 g/dL]
- Serum ferritin: 20 µg/dL [normal 50–200 µg/dL]
- Peripheral smear shows microcytic hypochromic picture

1. What is the probable diagnosis in this case?
2. What are the dietary sources rich in iron?

Explanation

This young lady is suffering with iron deficiency anemia. Iron is needed in ferrous form for synthesis of heme. Deficiency of iron impairs heme synthesis and results in hypochromic microcytic anemia.

In India, iron deficiency in female is a grave problem. Most of the time this is due to reduced dietary intake of iron. Iron-rich foods are green leafy vegetables, pulses, jaggery, etc. (Refer Fig. 34.4 above).

Case 2: A 10-year-old boy came to the OPD with complain of loss of appetite, early fatigue, lethargy. Mother complained that boy is soon tired and suffer from headache frequently. On examination, nails were flat and pallor was seen. Peripheral smear showed hypochromic, microcytic picture. Nails were brittle (Fig. 34.10).

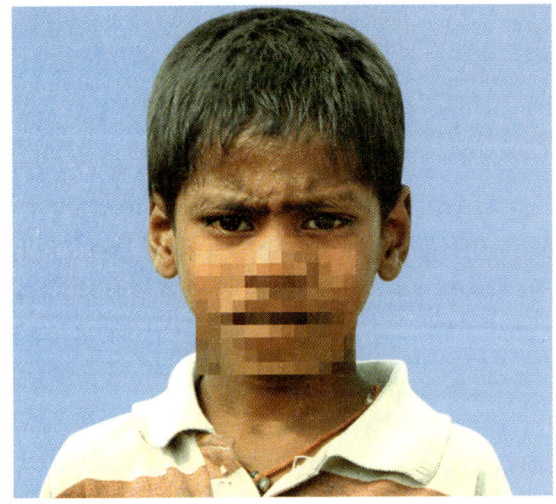

Fig. 34.10: Pale anemic child

1. What may be the probable diagnosis?
2. Which micronutrient is related with this disorder?
3. What other investigations you will plan to confirm the diagnosis?
4. What are the causes which will lead to this disorder?

Explanation

This child is suffering with iron deficiency anemia.

Investigations required are serum iron level, total iron binding capacity (TIBC), transferrin saturation.

In addition to dietary deficiency which is the major cause for iron deficiency anemia, hookworm infection, chronic loss through bleeding piles are important reason of iron deficiency anemia in Indian population.

Iodine Deficiency

A 26-year-old lady presents with complain of swelling in the neck for past 5 months which has been progressively increasing in size. She is giving the history of recent weight gain and lethargy and oligomenorrhea.

1. What may the cause of above manifestation?
2. What is diagnosis in this case?
3. Which micronutrient is responsible for such presentation?
4. What are all organs get affected in this disorder?

Explanation

This lady is having goitrous hypothyroidism which is due to deficiency of dietary iodine.

Iodine is required for synthesis of thyroid hormones T_3 and T_4. In deficiency of iodine intake, the thyroid gland enlarges due to proliferation of its follicle in an attempt to compensate thyroid hormone production and presents as multinodular goitre (MNG) (Fig. 34.11).

Treatment is iodine supplementation.

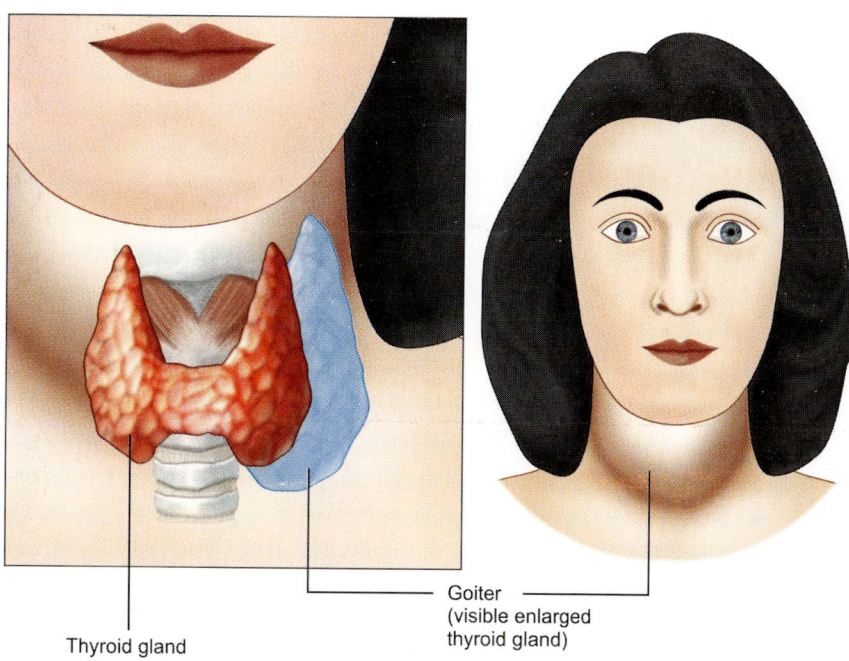

Fig. 34.11: Goiter

Acrodermatitis Enteropathica

A 2-year-old child bought to OPD with the history of irritability, stunted growth, diarrhea, loss of taste sensation, alopecia, and erythematous rashes over the face, perineum, and extremities (Fig. 34.12).

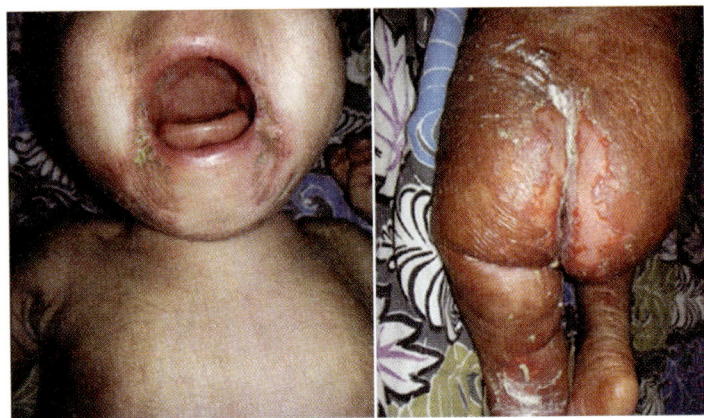

Fig. 34.12: Acrodermatitis enteropathica

Lesions over face and perineal area are typically symmetrical.
1. What may be the possible micronutrient deficiency in this baby?
2. What is the treatment advised?

Explanation

Baby may be suffering with the deficiency of zinc which is seen in 'acrodermatitis enteropathica' a rare autosomal recessive disorder, characterized by defective zinc absorption.

Treatment can be given by oral supplementation of elemental zinc (60 mg twice a day).

Toxicity of zinc may be seen in welding industries where workers are exposed to welding fumes. It is characterized by fever, respiratory distress, excessive salivation, headache and sweating.

Notes

Notes

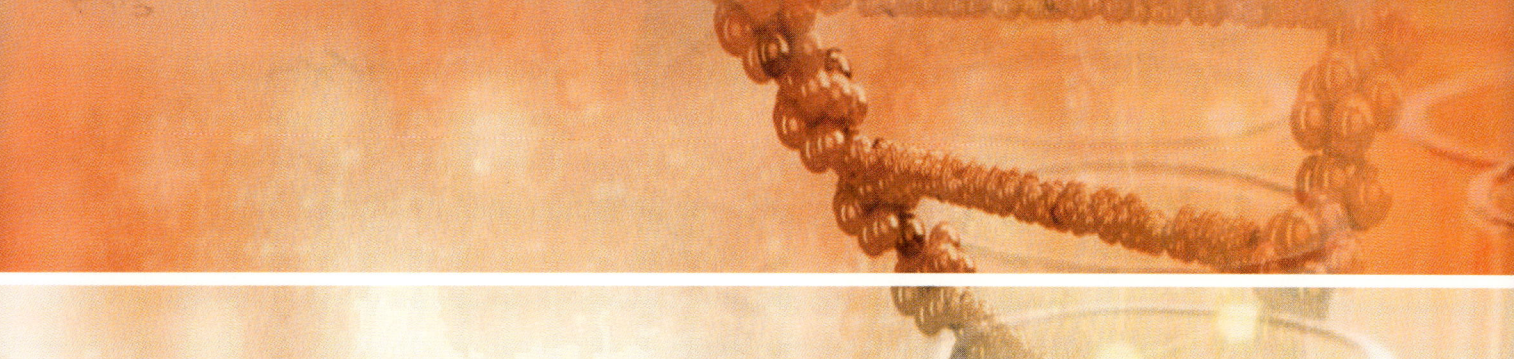

Section VII

Techniques

35. Electrophoresis
36. Chromatography

CHAPTER 35

Electrophoresis

Competency

PE 29.16: Discuss the indications for hemoglobin electrophoresis and interpret the report.

What is Electrophoresis?

Migration of charged solute or particle in a liquid medium under the influence of electric field is known as electrophoresis.

In this technique, charged components are separated based on their differential mobility in an electric field. The mobility in electrophoresis is based on charge-mass ratio.

Components of Electrophoresis (Fig. 35.1)

1. Support medium
2. Buffer
3. Power bank
4. Sample
5. Staining solution
6. Detection system

   Support media which are used are agarose gel, polyacrylamide gel, cellulose acetate, starch, etc.

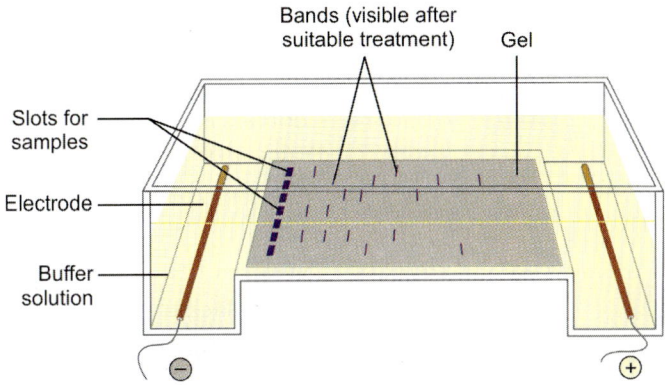

Fig. 35.1: Electrophoresis instrument

Functions of **buffer** ion are as follow:
a. Carry the applied current.
b. Fix the pH at which the electrophoresis is carried out.
c. Determine the status of charge on the solute.

Widely used buffer systems in electrophoresis are 'barbital buffer' and 'Tris-boric acid-EDTA buffer'.

Table 35.1 represents important **stains** which are being used for staining purpose.

What is the Principle of Electrophoresis?

Mobility on electrophoresis depends upon:
- Net charge on the molecule
- Size and shape of the particle
- Strength of electric field
- Physical and chemical characteristics of support medium
- Temperature of operation

How many types of electrophoresis is there?

Zonal Electrophoresis

Here charged macromolecules are separated in a porous support media like paper, agarose gel, starch gel, cellulose acetate, polyacrylamide, etc.

There are wide range of compounds which can be separated by zonal electrophoresis. They are:
1. Proteins
2. Hemoglobin
3. Lipoproteins
4. Isoenzymes
5. DNA fragments

1. Protein Electrophoresis

Serum, urinary, CSF protein can be measured using electrophoresis.

Gel which can be used for protein electrophoresis may be agarose gel or 7.5% polyacrylamide gel.

Table 35.1: Staining dye in various electrophoresis	
Separation type	*Stain*
Serum protein	Amido Black Coomassie Brilliant Blue G-250 Coomassie Brilliant Blue R-250 Ponceau-S
Isoenzymes	Nitro tetrazolium blue
Lipoprotein	Fat red 7B Oil red O Sudan black B
DNA fragments	Ethidium bromide
CSF proteins	Silver nitrate

In a normal serum, total five bands are seen (Table 35.2):
1. Albumin
2. Alpha-1 (α-1)
3. Alpha-2 (α-2)
4. Beta (β)
5. Gamma (γ)

Sixth band may be seen in fresh serum or if calcium is present in buffer.
Densitometer is used for quantification of each band.

Following clinical conditions result in abnormal bands (Fig. 35.2):
- Nephrotic syndrome: Decreased albumin and γ band
- Chronic infection, cirrhosis: Fusion of beta and gamma band
- Multiple myeloma: An unusual band called M band is seen in γ region which is because of IgA monoclonal gammopathy.

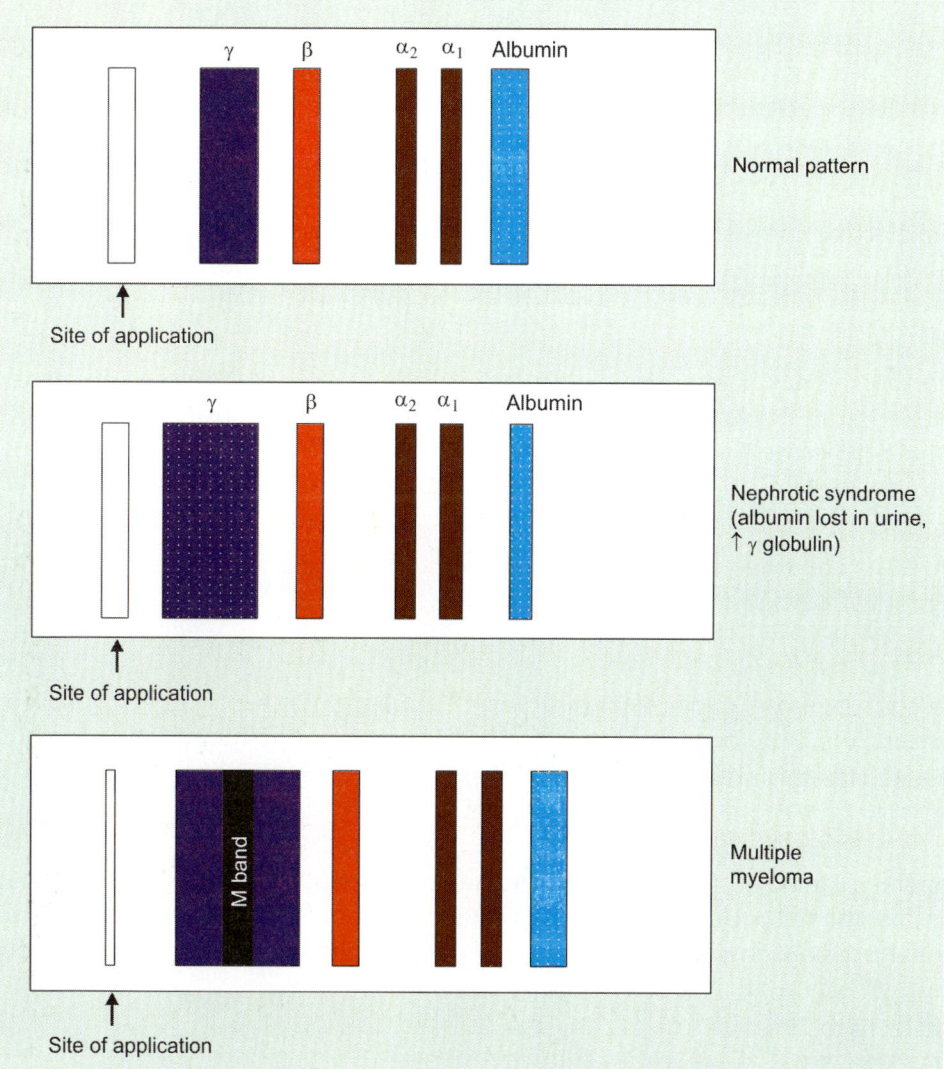

Fig. 35.2: Protein EPP in different disease states

Table 35.2: Composition of proteins in different electrophoretic regions in a serum electrophoresis		
Electrophoretic band	Percentage in a normal serum	Proteins
Albumin	55–65%	Albumin
Alpha-1 (α-1)	2–4%	α-1 antitrypsin α-1 glycoprotein α-1 fetoprotein
Alpha-2 (α-2)	6–12%	α-2 macroglobulin Ceruloplasmin Haptoglobin
Beta (β)	8–12%	Transferrin β2 microglobulin C3 C4
Gamma (γ)	12–22%	IgG IgA IgM C-reactive protein

2. Hemoglobin Electrophoresis

Hemoglobin electrophoresis is used to find out abnormal hemoglobin like HbS, HbC, Hb variants like HbF and also derived hemoglobin HbA1c. They are separated by cellulose acetate electrophoresis due to their different mobility on electrophoretic plate compared to normal adult hemoglobin (HbA).

Hb electrophoresis for diagnosis of sickle cell trait and sickle cell disease: In alkaline medium (pH 8.6), HbS migrates slower compared to HbA towards anode (positive electrode). This is due to the fact that replacement of glutamate by valine at 6th position of beta chain in HbS reduces the electronegativity on HbS and it results in slower movement of HbS towards anode (Fig. 35.3).

Hb electrophoresis for separation of glycated hemoglobin (HbA1) from unglycated hemoglobin (HbA0): HbA0 has retarded migration as compared to HbA1 due to greater interaction of charged group of agars with HbA0 (Fig. 35.4).

3. Lipoprotein Electrophoresis

Cellulose acetate, agarose, paper electrophoresis can be used to separate various lipoproteins by electrophoresis. It is more of a qualitative method than being the quantitative method.

This helps in classification of dyslipoproteinemia (Fig. 35.5).

4. Isoenzyme Electrophoresis

LDH isoenzymes can be separated using agarose gel or cellulose acetate electrophoresis at pH of 6.3. During this, the LDH-1 moves the fastest on electrophoresis and LDH-5 moves the least (Fig. 35.6). It is quantitated using densitometer. Following are the percentages of LDH isoenzyme in a normal healthy individual:

- LDH-1(H4): 14 to 26%
- LDH-2(H3 M1): 29 to 39%
- LDH-3(H2M2): 20 to 26%

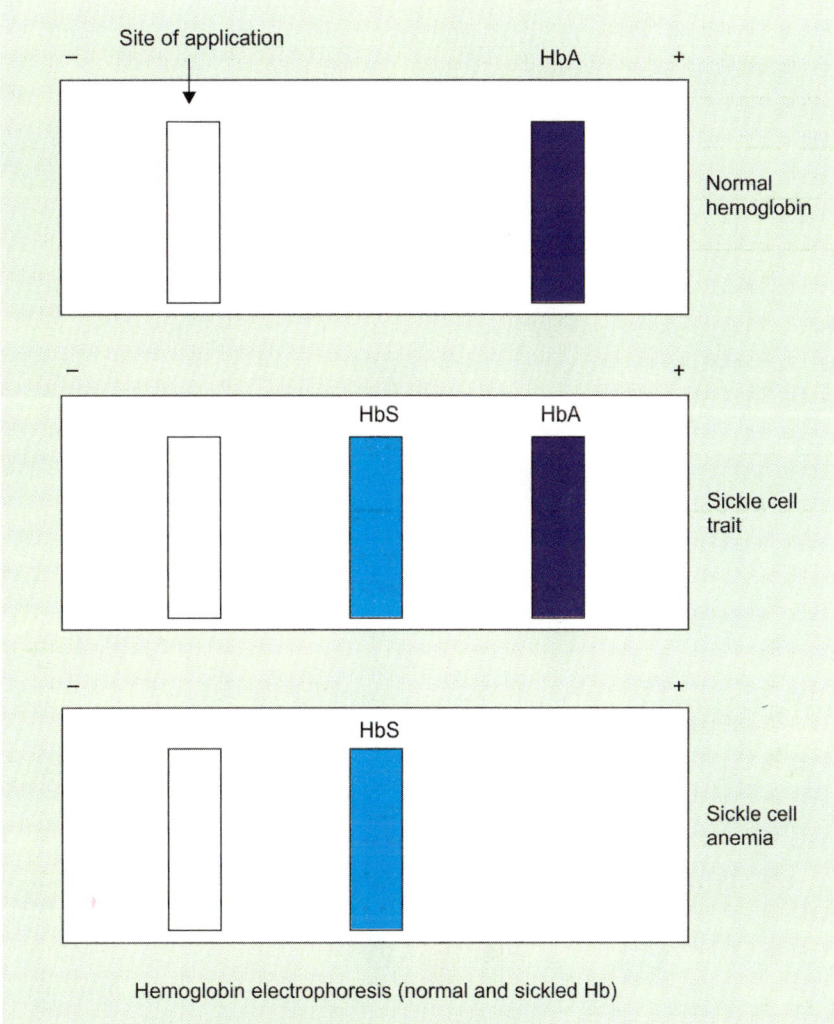

Fig. 35.3: EPP band in HbS

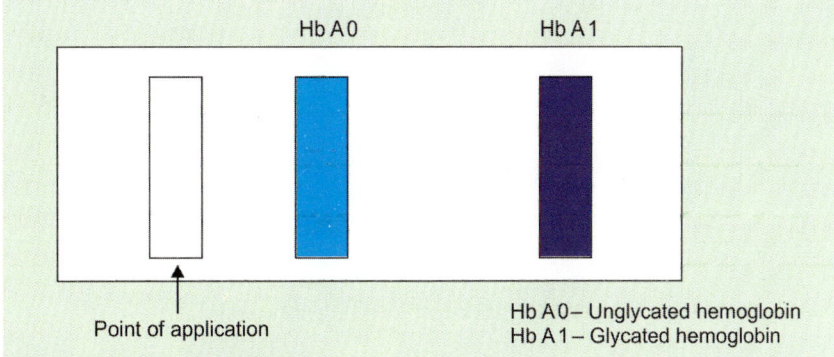

Fig. 35.4: EPP band for HbA0 and HbA1

- LDH-4(H1M3): 8 to 16%
- LDH-5(H4): 6 to 16%

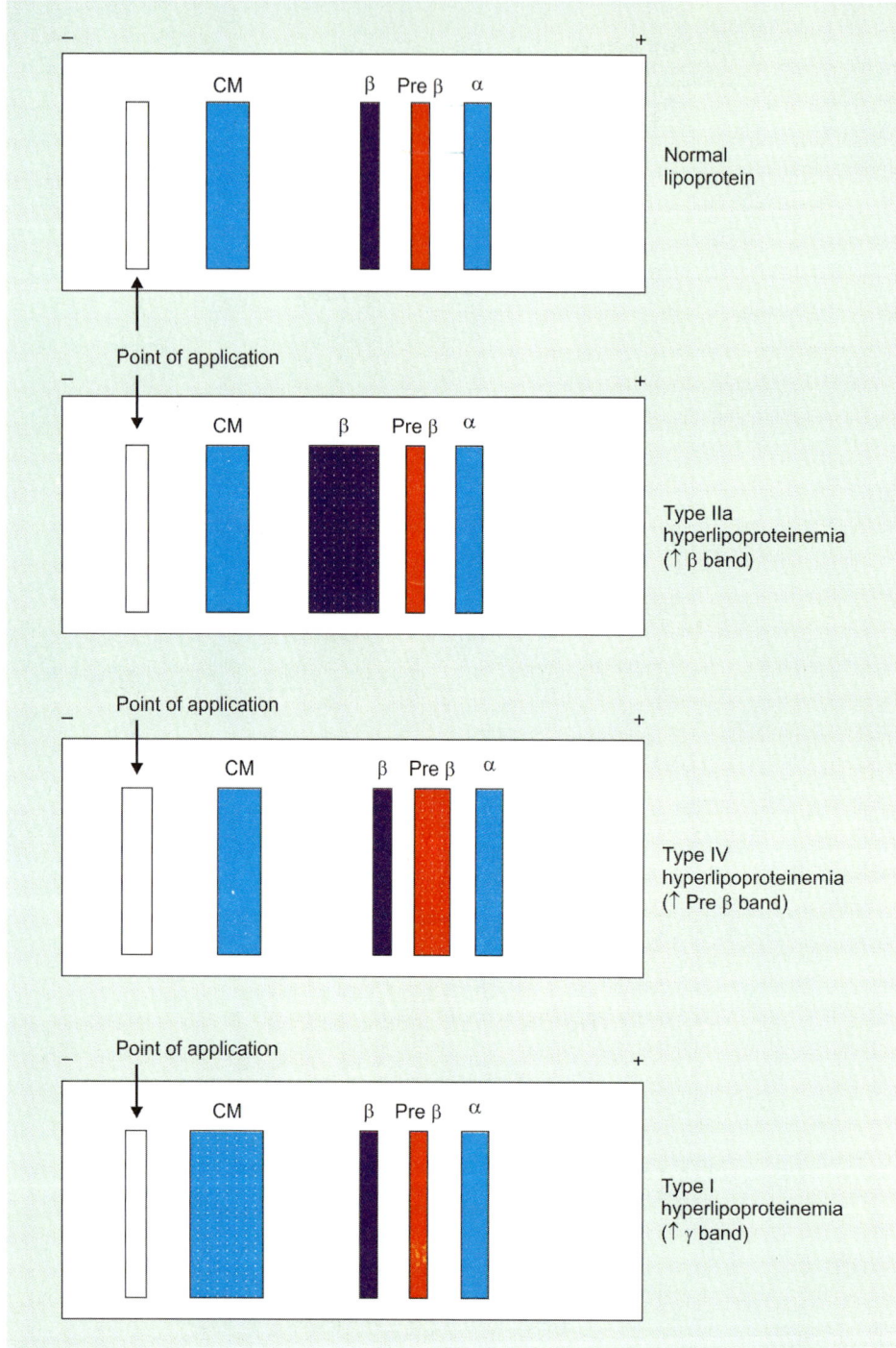

Fig. 35.5: Lipoprotein electrophoresis

In a normal healthy individual, LDH-2 is more than LDH-1, and their ratio is 0.45 to 0.74.

In case of myocardial infarction, LDH-1 becomes more than LDH-2 due to leakage of LDH-1 from heart tissues. This pattern of reversal of LDH ratio is known as **flipped pattern of LDH** which is an important finding in myocardial infarction.

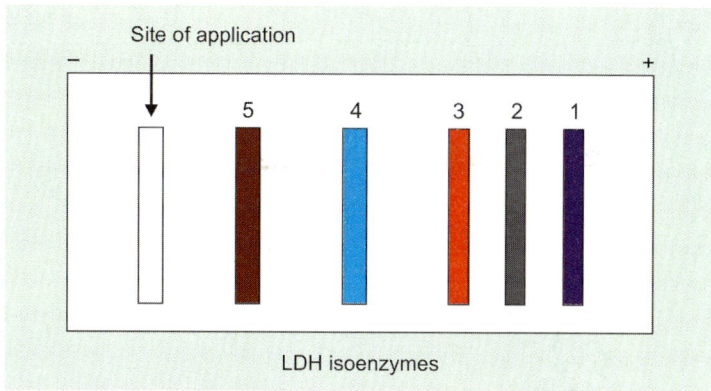

Fig. 35.6: LDH isoenzymes on EPP

5. DNA Fragment Electrophoresis

DNA and RNA have evenly distributed negative charge and hence they tend to move under electric field and get separated. Mostly the gel used for DNA/RNA electrophoresis is agarose gel electrophoresis.

Ethidium bromide is mixed in the gel which is used for DNA electrophoresis and it intercalates the adjacent bases in the nucleic acid and is visible under UV transillumination.

Isoelectric Focusing (IEF)

Here the stable pH gradient is used on the support medium. The amphoteric compounds like proteins are then separated based on their isoelectric pH(pI) (Fig. 35.7).

Proteins differing in their isoelectric pH value of only 0.02 can be separated using IEF.

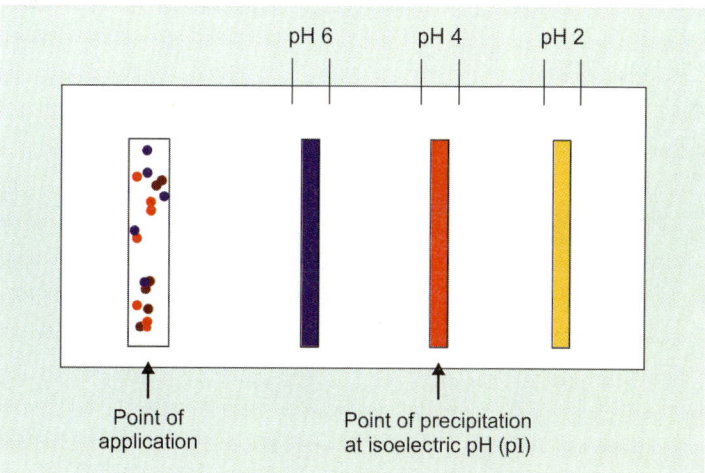

Fig. 35.7: Isoelectric focusing

Two-Dimensional Electrophoresis

Here electrophoresis is done in two directions. First the electrophoresis is done in one direction based on charge mass (size) ratio. Then the slide is treated with sodium dodecyl sulfate to neutralize the charge. This is followed by electrophoresis in other direction where only size is taken into consideration (Fig. 35.8).

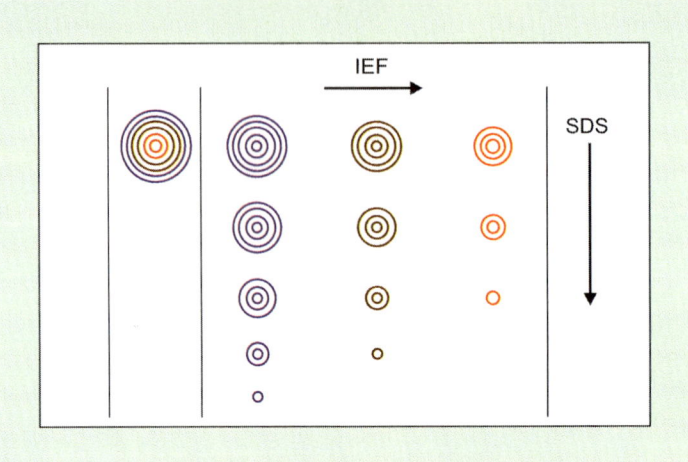

Fig. 35.8: Two-dimensional electrophoresis

Capillary Electrophoresis

Here the electrophoresis is done in capillary lumen.

Advantages:
a. Small volume of sample required
b. Quick to process
c. Ease of automation

Notes

CHAPTER 36

Chromatography

> **Competency**
>
> **BI 11.5:** Describe screening of urine for inborn errors and describe the use of paper chromatography.

Chromatography is the technique which is used to separate the components of a mixture based on their diverse physical characteristics (Fig. 36.1).

The differential interaction of the compounds of a mixture between stationary and mobile phases helps in separation of these compounds using suitable set of stationary and mobile phases.

Important components of any chromatography technique are:
1. Stationary phase
2. Mobile phase
3. Platform which holds the stationary phase (column or paper).
4. Mixture, the components of which need to be separated.

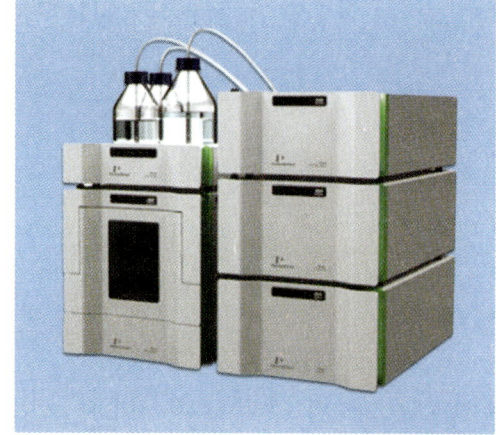

Fig. 36.1: Chromatography instrument

Stationary phase may be solid, liquid or rarely gas, but mobile phase may be either liquid or gas alone.

Based on physical characteristic which is used to separate the components of a mixture, following types of chromatography are designed:
1. Size exclusion chromatography (stearic exclusion/gel chromatography)
2. Ion exchange chromatography
3. Partition chromatography
4. Adsorption chromatography

Size Exclusion Chromatography
(Stearic Exclusion/Gel Filtration/Gel Permeation Chromatography)

In this type of chromatography, porous material is packed in the column, pore size of which is selected based on the size of molecule being separated, and the mixture containing varied size of particles is mixed in mobile phase and poured over the stationary column (Fig. 36.2).

Chromatography

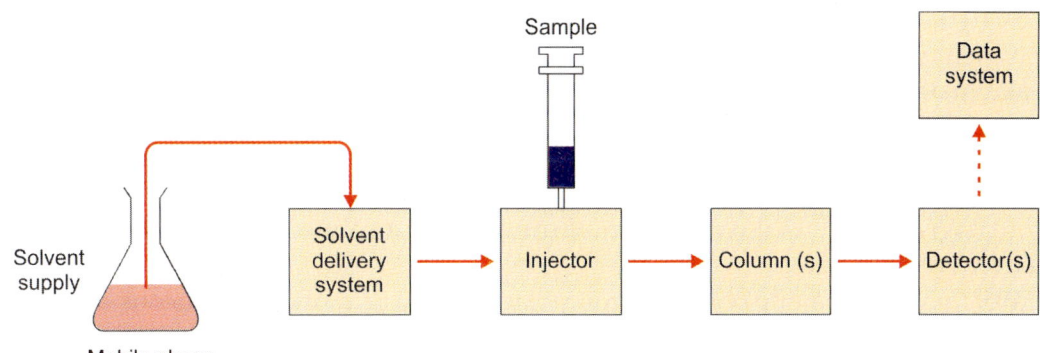

Fig. 36.2: Schematic diagram of chromatography

Those molecules, the size of which corresponds to the internal diameter of porous material, are trapped in the pores transiently and move the slowest. Larger molecules are permeating through steric exclusion and move out the fastest (Fig. 36.3).

Presently silica or glass materials are selected to design the beads for column packing.

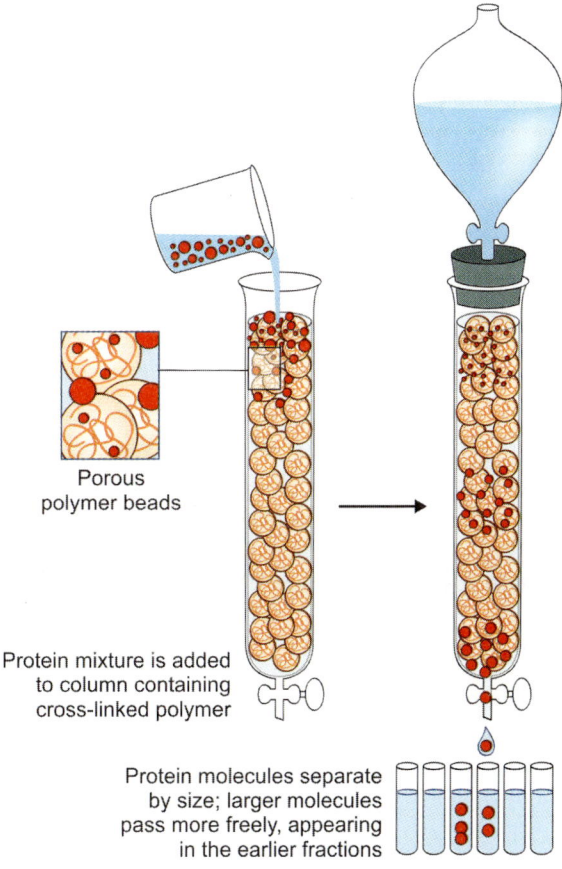

Fig. 36.3: Size exclusion chromatography

Ion Exchange Chromatography

In this type of chromatography, components of the mixture are separated based on their charge. Stationary column is packed with resins having the charge on it.

In cation exchange chromatography, stationary phase is packed with the resin having negative charge on them which holds back the positive ions (cations), and in anion exchange chromatography, stationary phase is packed with the resin having positive charge on them which holds back the negative ions (anions).

Partition Chromatography

This chromatography is based on differential solubility of a solute between polar (aqueous) and non-polar (organic) solvents.

Mixture of molecules having polar and non-polar groups is dissolved in aqueous solvent (mobile phase) and is poured over the organic solvent (stationary phase).

Polar molecules remain in aqueous medium and non-polar compounds are dissolved in organic solvent; hence, they are separated.

Adsorption Chromatography

It is an obsolete type of chromatography which is based on the relative affinity (adsorption capacity) of solute between mobile and stationary phases.

Types of chromatography based on platform at which stationary media are allocated:
1. *Column chromatography*: Stationary media are filled in a column.
2. *Thin layer chromatography*: Thin layer of silica gel, cellulose, alumina, cross-linked dextran is layer over the glass or plastic plate.
   - Sample is applied on one end and this plate is kept in solvent which is the mobile phase. Chromatographic chamber which is already saturated with solvent vapor is used for the purpose.
   - Solvent ascends the plate through capillary action taking the sample along with it.
   - Retention factor is calculated by following formula:

$$R_f = \text{Distance travelled by solute/Distance travelled by solvent}$$

Experiment

Here the process used in paper chromatography is described.

Material Required

1. Whatman filter paper no 1
2. Solvent: n-butanol: acetic acid: distilled water (12:3:5)
3. Amino acid solution
4. Test tube with diameter 1 cm
5. Capillaries for sample application
6. Ninhydrin mixture (0.1%)
7. Pencil
8. Cotton balls

Steps (Fig. 36.4)

Gloves should be worn to handle the chromatography paper to avoid the skin mark artifacts on the paper.

1. In a test tube, 2 mL of solvent should be taken and it should be plugged with cotton ball as to saturate the atmosphere.

Chromatography

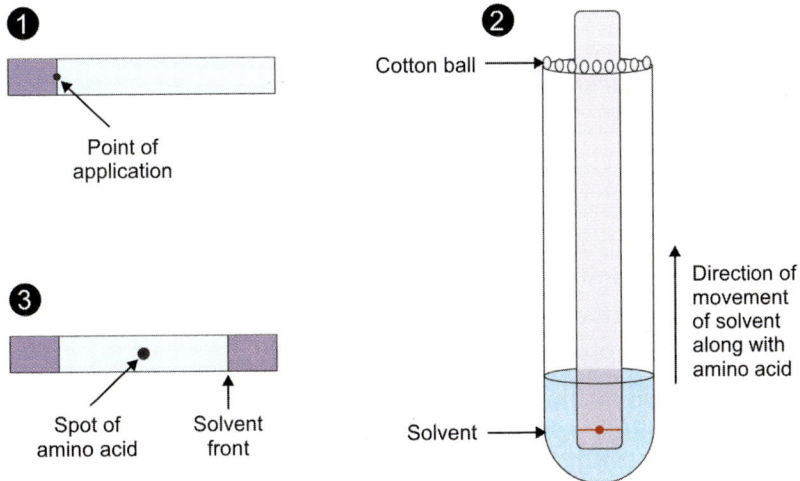

Fig. 36.4: Steps for doing chromatography in UG lab

2. After this, 15 cm × 1.5 cm strips of paper are cut. (Width of the paper should be according to diameter of the test tube being used.)
3. A line is drawn with pencil 2.5 cm above one edge.
4. In the center of this line, amino acid mixture is applied with the help of capillary tube. Two to three drops may suffice. After applying each drop, it should be dried properly by putting the paper in hot air oven.
5. Paper is kept carefully in the test tube in a fashion that marked line is little above the solvent layer and TT should be capped with cotton ball.
6. Care should be taken that paper is not touching the wall of the glass tube.
7. The test tube is left as such for 30–40 minutes time or till the time the solvent front is seen to reach near the upper end of the tube.
8. Strip is removed at this time solvent front is marked with pencil and this strip is kept in hot air oven at 100°C for 10 min.
9. Ninhydrin solution is sprayed on it to completely cover the paper and once again it is kept in hot air oven to dry.
10. Appearance of purple spot is noticed after the paper is dried.
11. Distance of solute movement from the point of sample application line is measured with scale and this distance is used as numerator of formula for R_f value.
12. Distance of solvent front from the point of sample application line is measured with scale and this distance is used as denominator of formula for R_f value.
13. R_f value is calculated by formula:

$$R_f = \text{Distance travelled by solute/Distance travelled by solvent}$$

R_f value obtained is compared with the documented values and the amino acid is identified.

VIVA VOCE

Q1. What is chromatography?

Ans. Chromatography is the technique which is used to separate the components of a mixture based on their diverse physical characteristics.

The differential interaction of the compounds of a mixture between stationary and mobile phases helps in separation of these compounds using suitable set of stationary and mobile phase.

Q2. What are all types of chromatography you know?

Ans. Based on physical characteristic which is used to separate the components of a mixture, following types of chromatography are designed:
1. Size exclusion chromatography (stearic exclusion/gel chromatography)
2. Ion exchange chromatography
3. Partition chromatography
4. Adsorption chromatography

Q3. What is R_f value?

Ans. R_f = Distance travelled by solute/Distance travelled by solvent

Based on R_f value, the amino acid is identified.

Q4. What paper is suitable for doing the chromatography?

Ans. Whatman filter paper no 1.

Q5. What are stationary and mobile phases of chromatography?

Ans. Mobile phase is the one which carries the mixture which is to be separated along with it and stationary phase is the medium over which the mobile phase is poured so that components of mixture interact with the stationary phase at varied capacity and get separated.

Stationary phase may be solid, liquid or rarely gas, but mobile phase may be either liquid or gas.

Notes

Notes